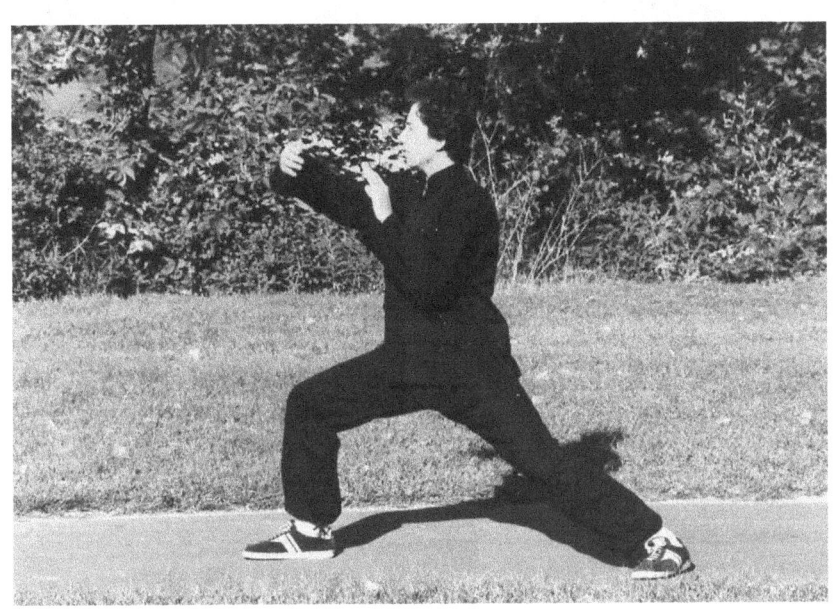

Harmony in Motion

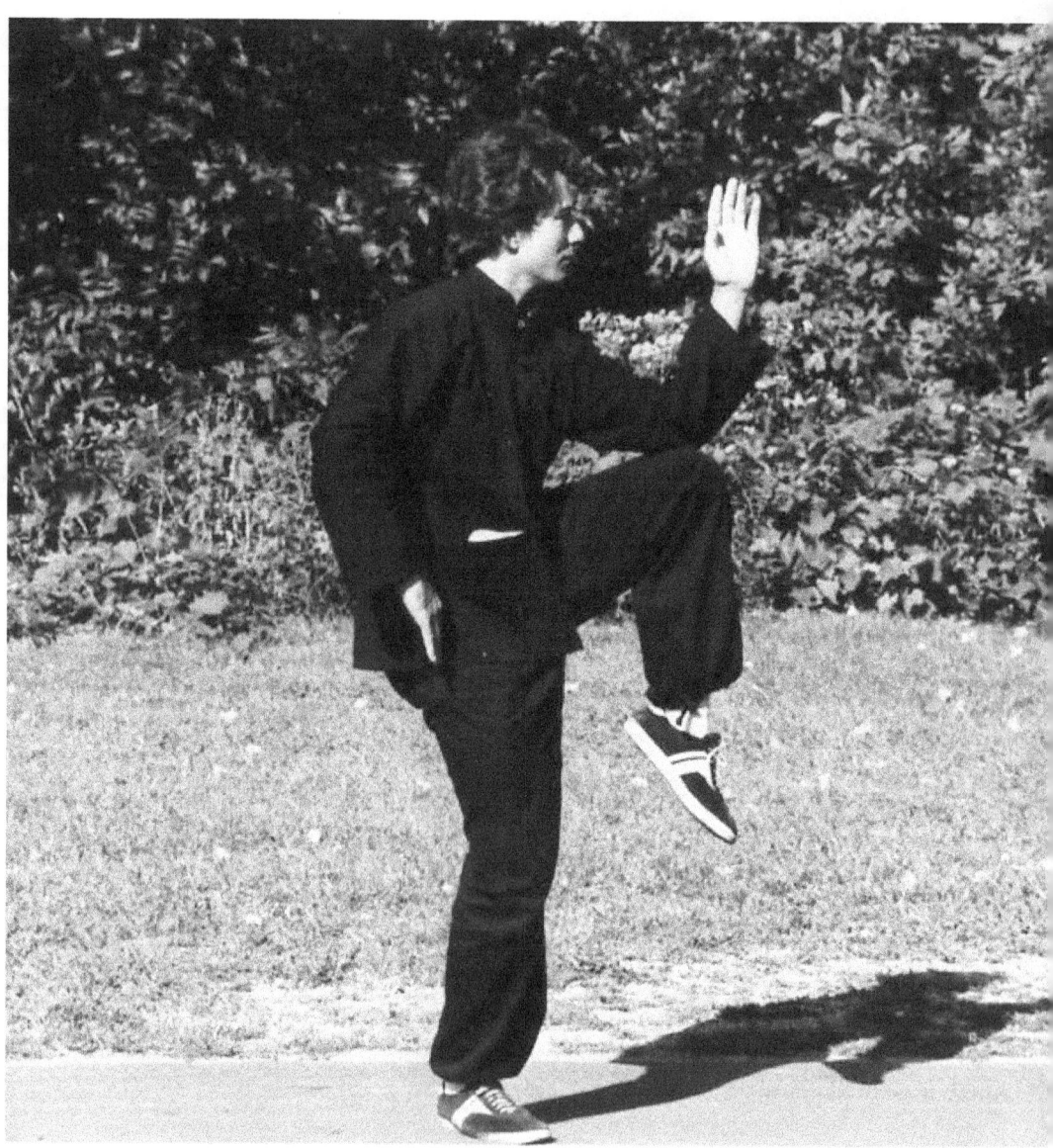

Harmony in Motion

Celebrating 40 years
of Sifu Ray Hayward's Taiji in Minnesota

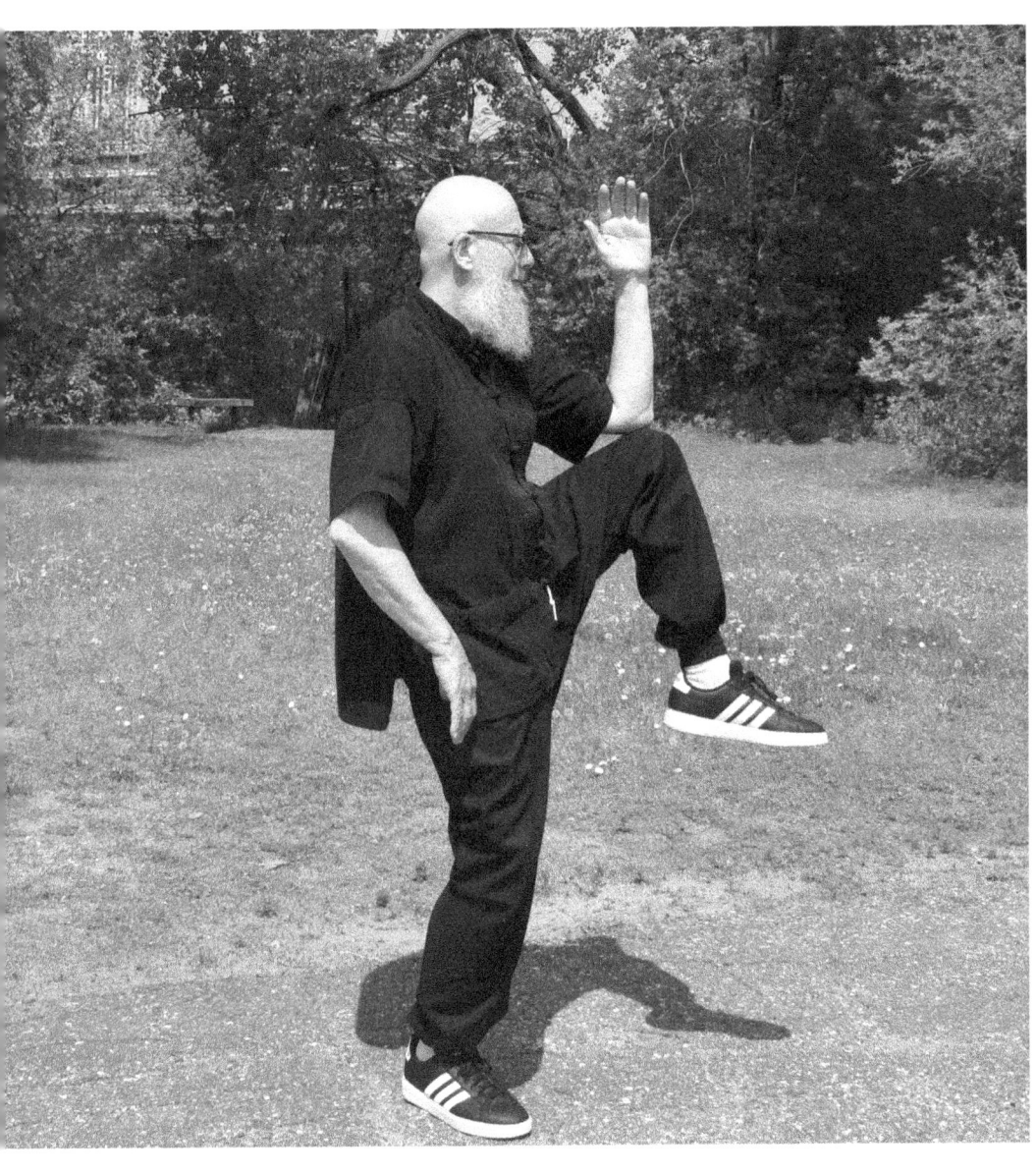

Compiled and edited by Margo Bock and Julie Cisler

Ray Hayward Enterprises

Harmony in Motion: Celebrating 40 years of Sifu Ray Hayward's Taiji in Minnesota

© Copyright 2024 by Ray Hayward. All rights reserved. No part of this book may be reproduced or circulated in any manner whatsoever without written permission from the author.

Photographs courtesy of Dan Dale, Dan Polsfus, Rose Davis, Robert Wozniac, Margo Bock, Julie Cisler, Wanda Koehler, Jerry Dewees, Fredrick Sparks, J. Richard Roy, Ray Hayward, Diane Cannon, Paul Ittner, John Feeley, Rondi Atkin, Michael Sauter, Bryan Davis, Michelle Ashmin, Bob Klanderud, Michael Cain, and Michael Newman.

Published by: Ray Hayward Productions
5140 W 102nd Street, #307
Bloomington, MN 55437
United States of America
(651) 271-3500

Disclaimer: The author and publisher of this book are not responsible for any injury that may result from following the instructions contained herein. The reader should consult his or her physician for advice before attempting any such activities.

ISBN 978-0-578-76315-6
1 2 3 4 5 6 / 29 28 27 26 25 24

Table of Contents

Masters Gallery. 6
Acknowledgements. 18

The Seventh Generation Speaks 19
Daniel Dale 21
Margo Bock 22
Jerry DeWees 23
Matthew Barrett 24
Paul Ittner 25
Wanda Koehler 27
John Feeley 28
Michelle Ashmun 30
Robert Wozniac 32
John Stitely 33
Rondi Atkin 36
Dominick Veldman 38
Michael Sauter 41
Christopher Venaccio 44
Karen Barton 46
Martin Ebelhardt 48
Sharon Nyberg 51
Michael Cain 52
Karen Deley 57
Julie Cisler 58
Diane Cannon 60
Frederick Sparks 64
Robert "Bob" Klanderud .66
James Postiglione 67
Bryan Davis 68

Sifu Speaks 70
Introduction to 40th Anniversary Book 71
5 Willows 78
Photo Essay 106

Appendix 114
Why You Should Study T'ai-Chi 115
Push Hands: Just One Aspect of Self-Defense 117
Yang Style Taijiquan Lineage 121
Joanne Von Blon: 1924-2024 122
About the Authors 123
Contact Information 126

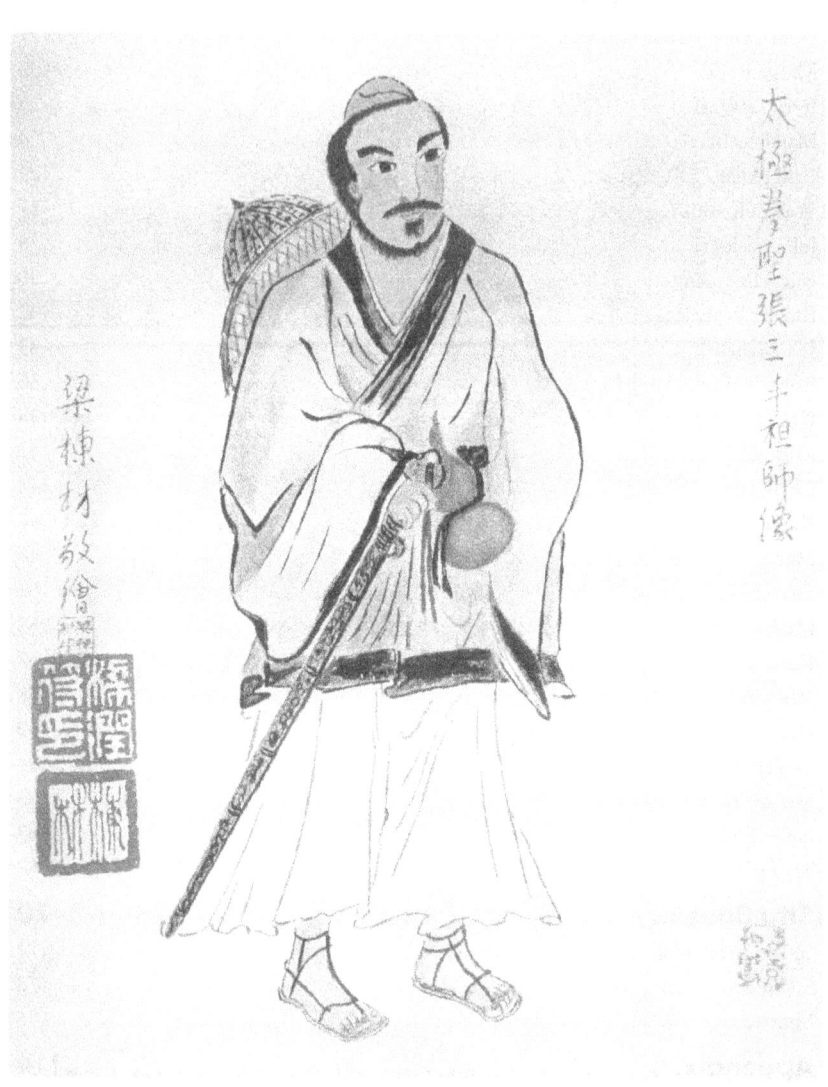

Zhang Sanfeng (張三丰)
Painting by T.T. Liang © 1980

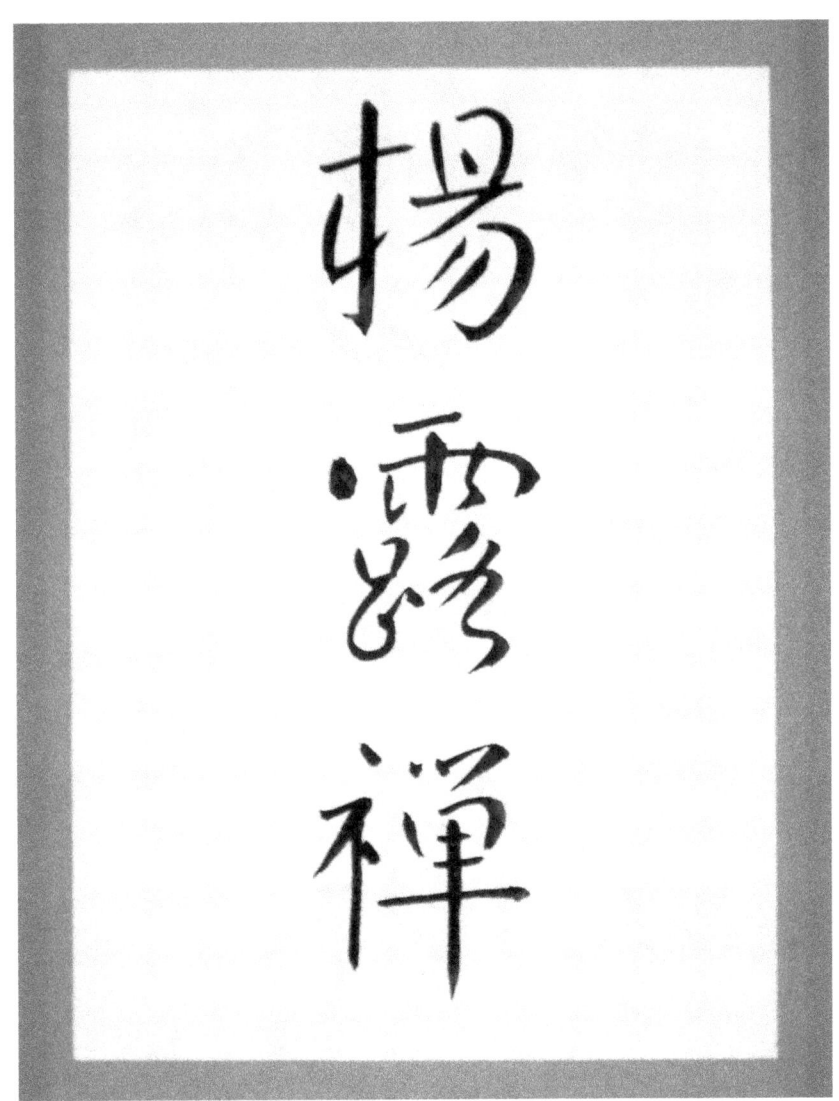

Yang Luchan (杨露禅)
Calligraphy by T.T. Liang

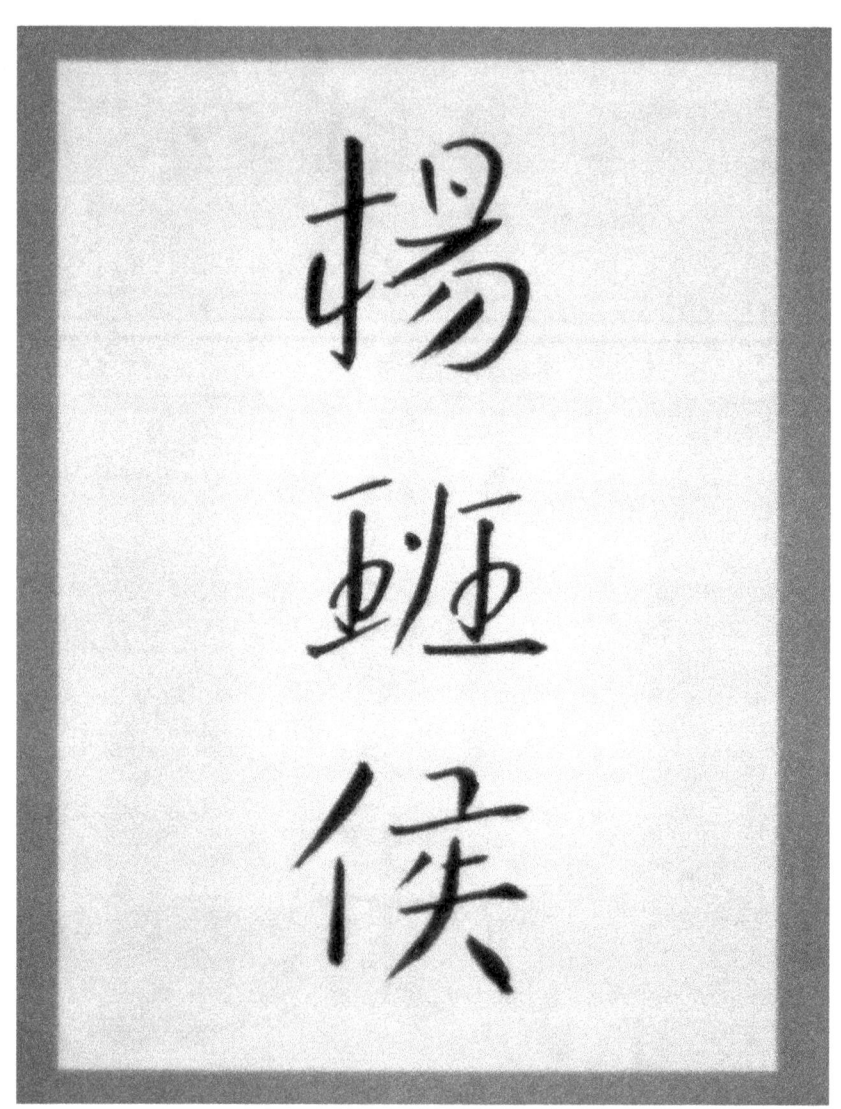

Yang Banhou (楊班侯)
Calligraphy by T.T. Liang

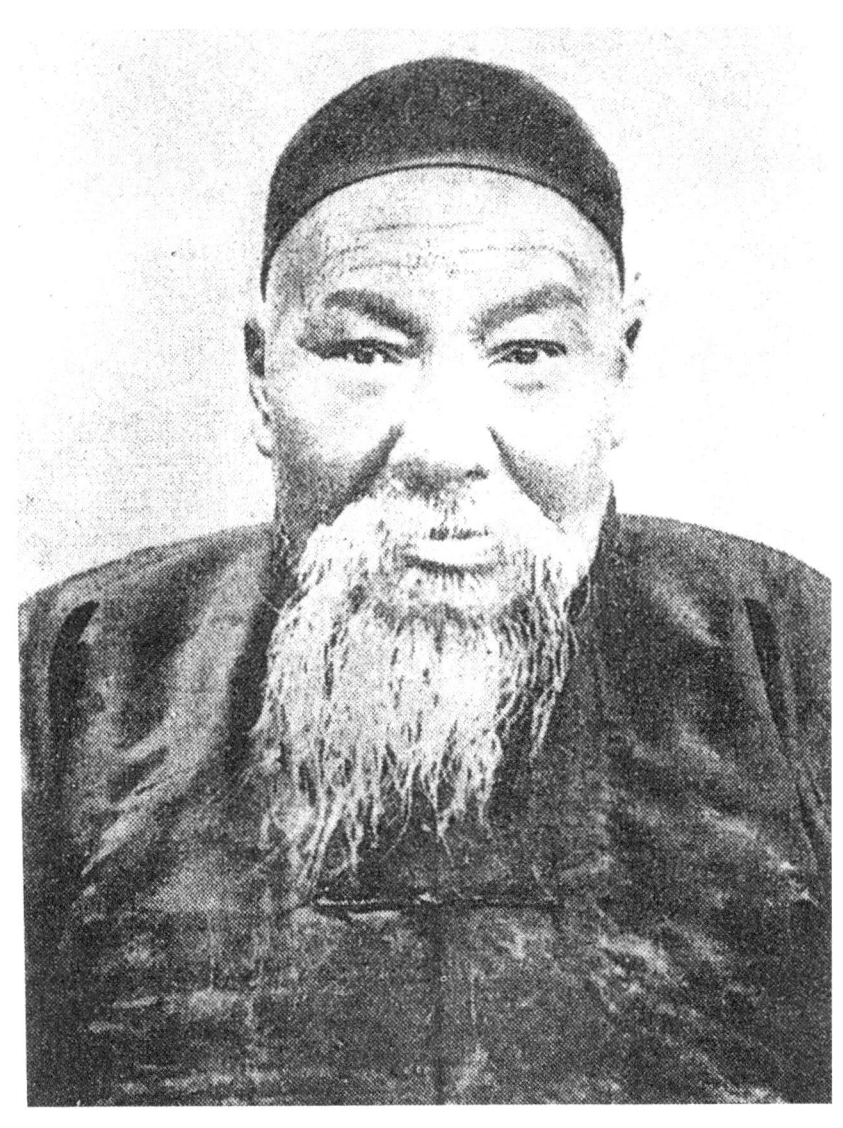

Yang Jianhou (楊健侯)

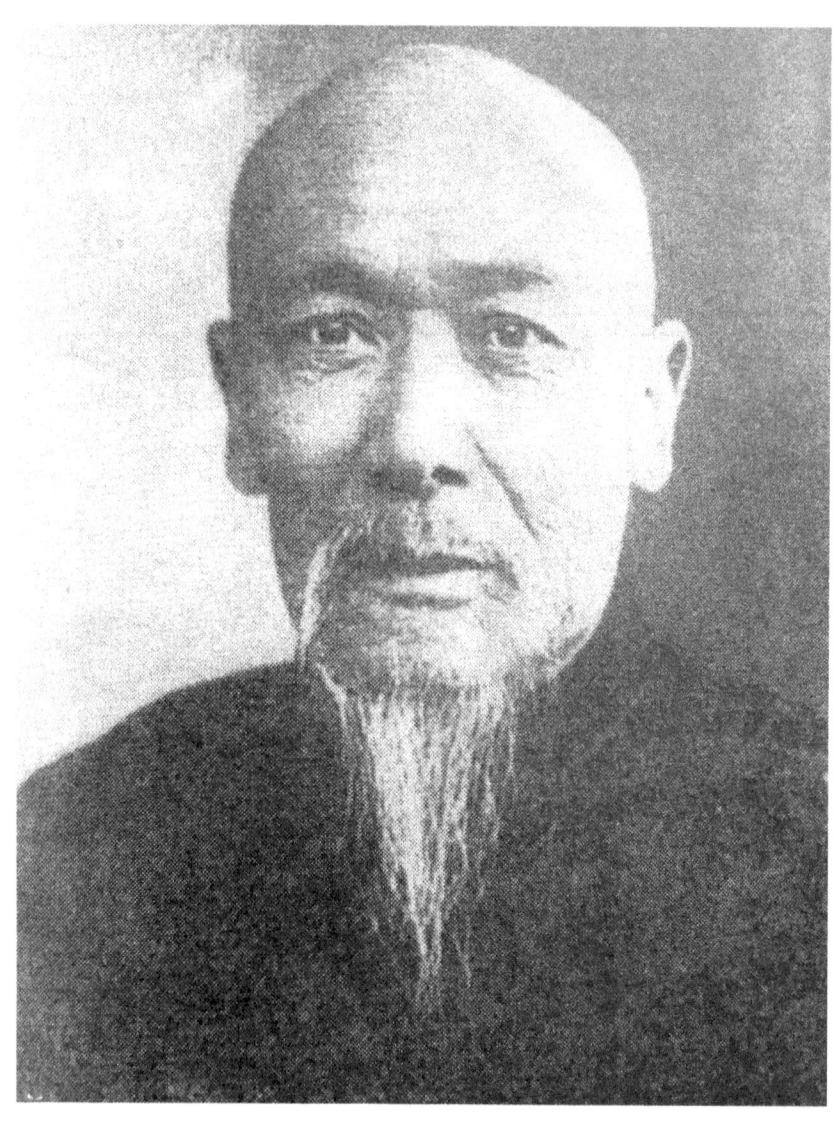

Yang Shaohou (楊少侯)

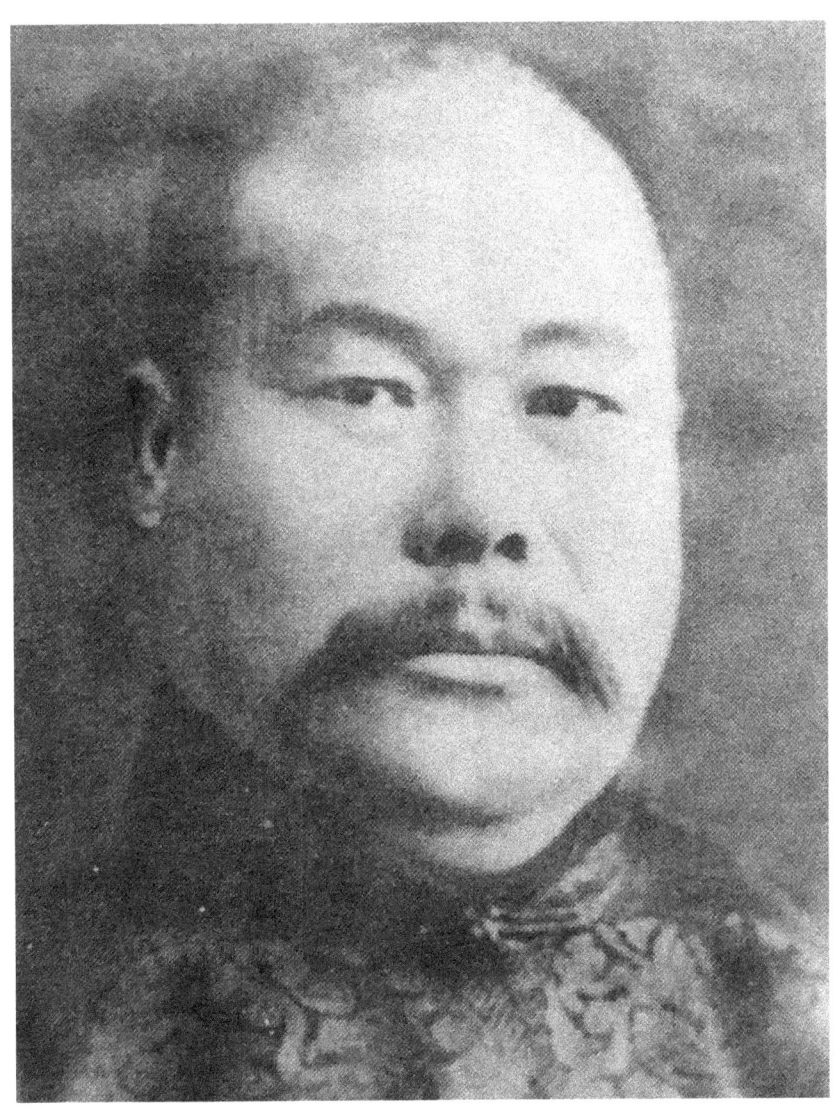

Yang Chengfu (杨澄甫)

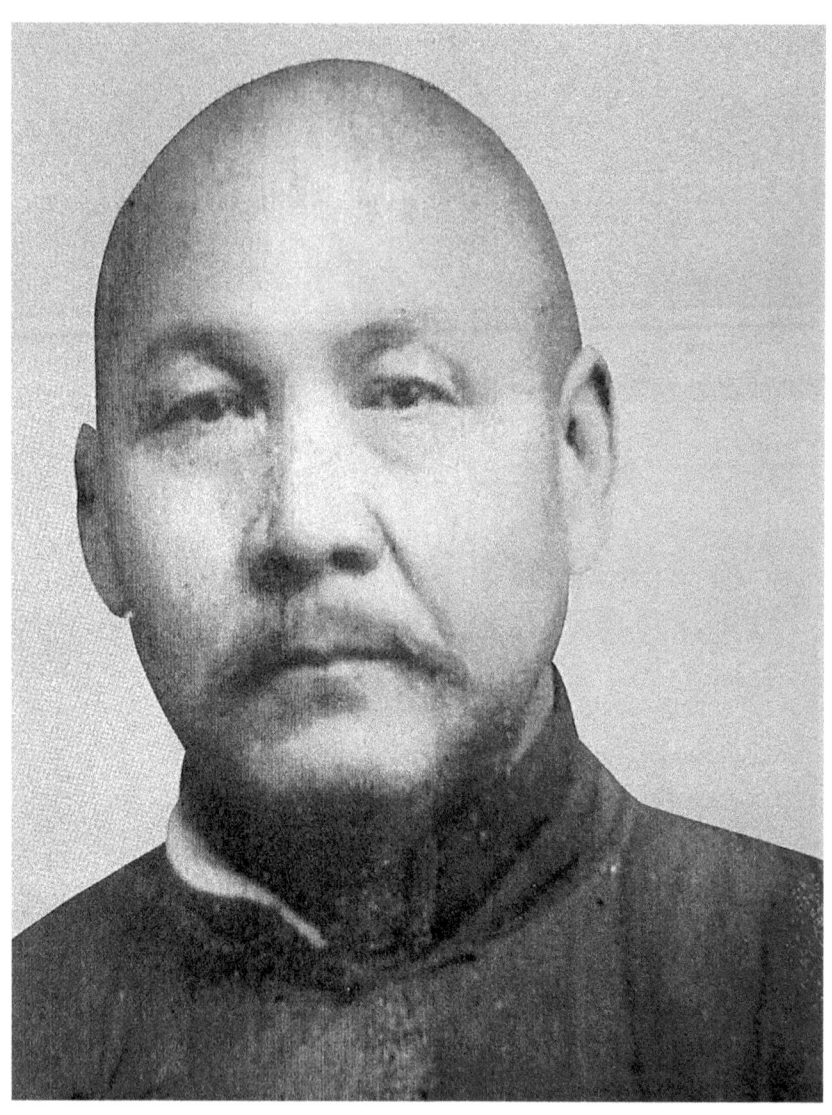

Zhang Qinlin (張欽霖)

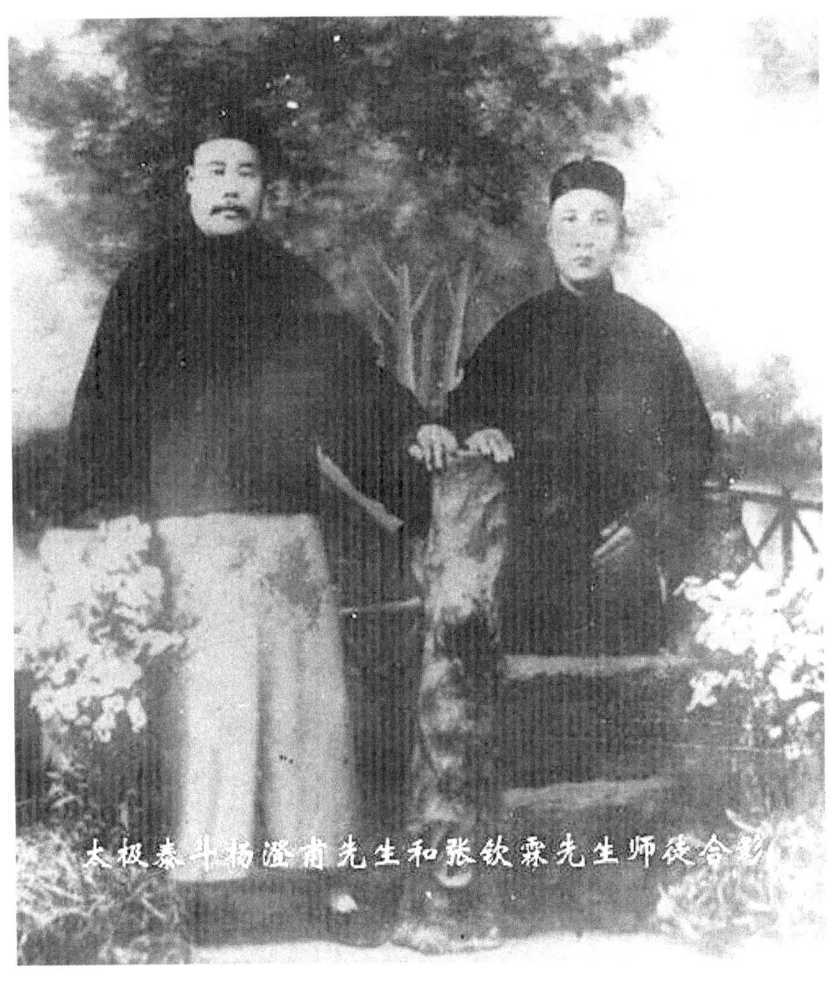

Yang Chengfu (*left*) and Zhang Qinlin (*right*)

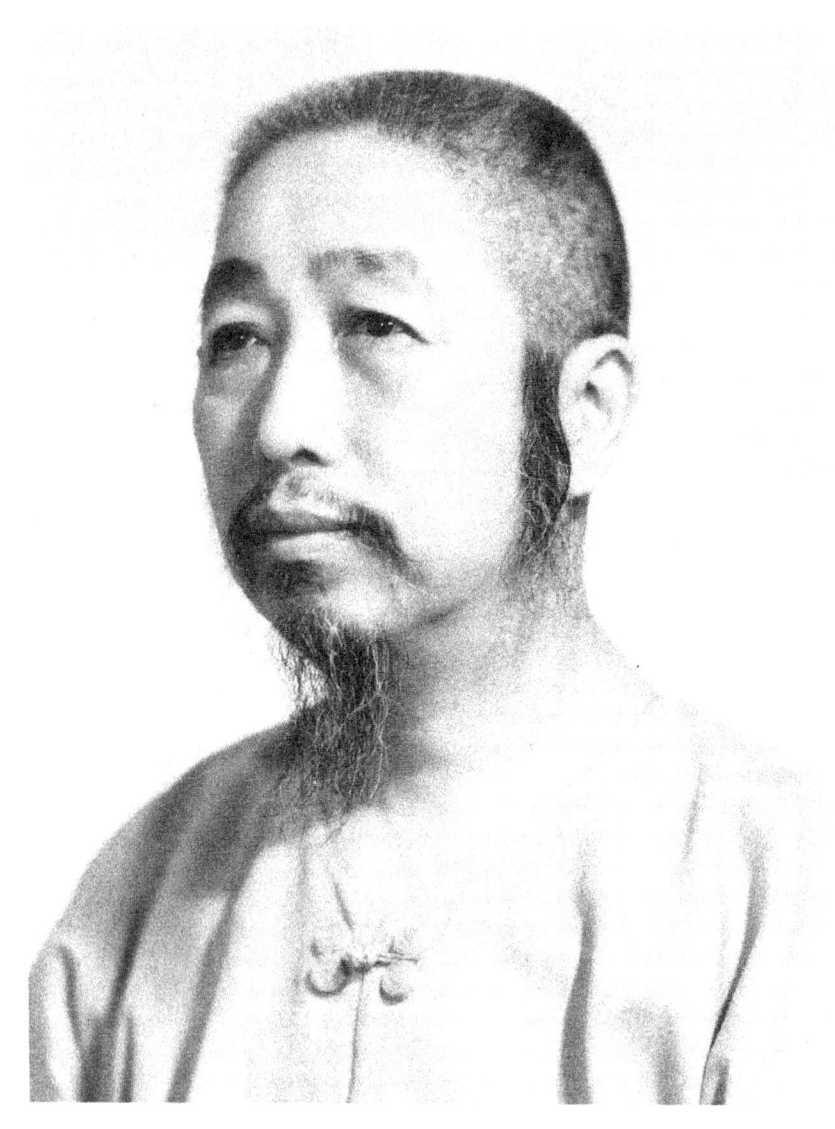

Zheng Manqing (郑曼青)

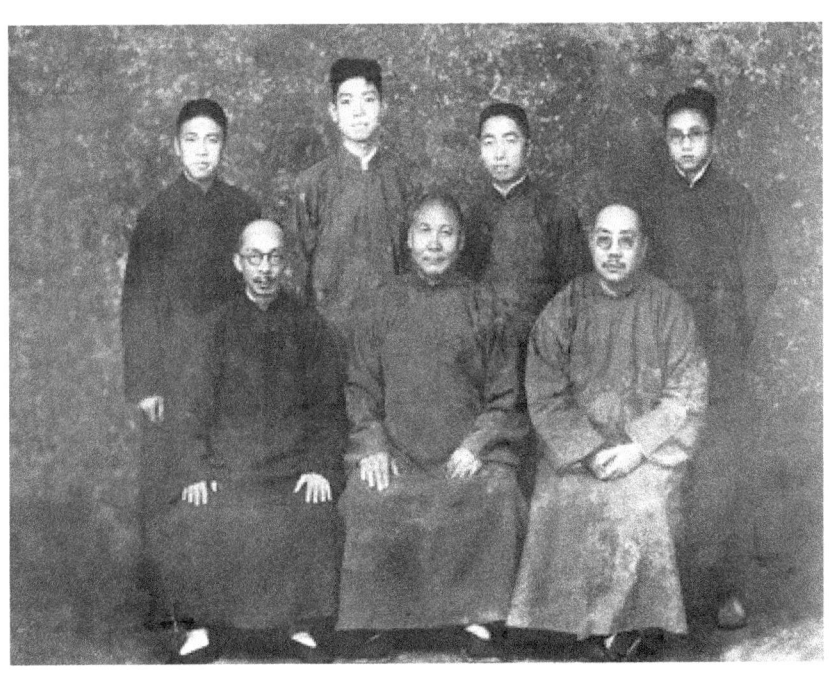

Zhang Qinlin (*front center*) and Zheng Manqing (*back second from right*)

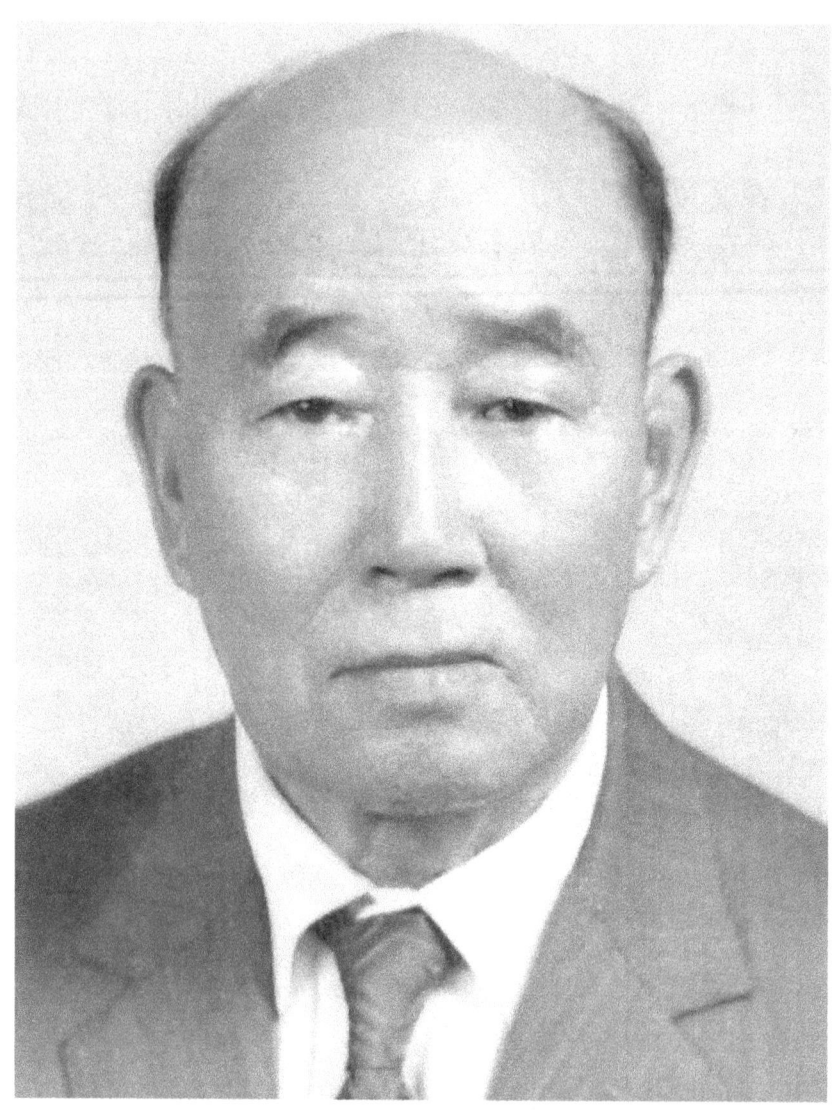

Liang Tungtsai (梁棟材)

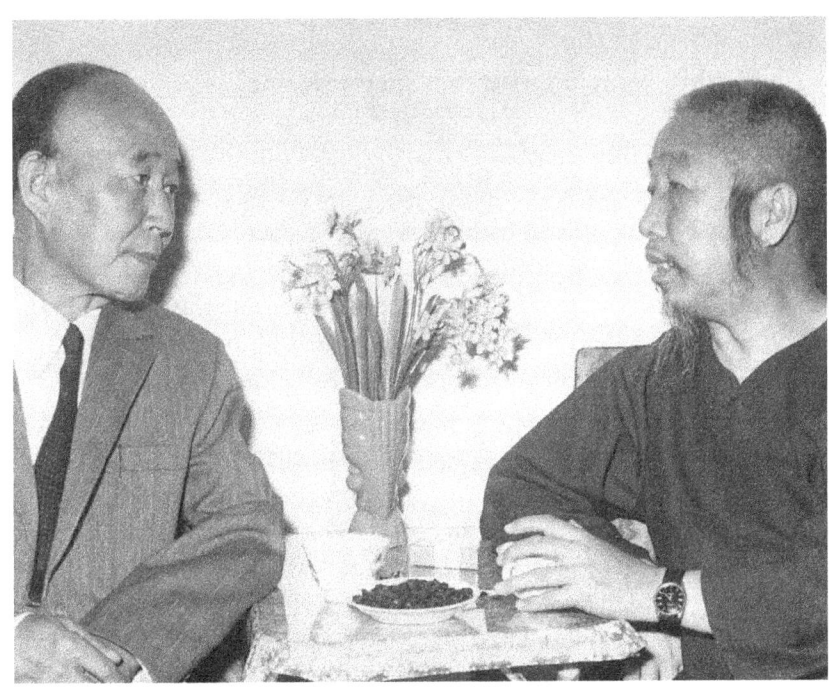

Zheng Manqing with Liang Tungtsai

Acknowledgements

To Dad, thank you for being a Golden Rooster Standing on One Leg at the right moment.

To Mark, thank you for supporting my Taiji journey and endeavors all these years.

~ Margo Bock

To my first Sifu, Richard Mesmer, for guiding the way for me to discover my love of Taiji.

To Matthew, for your patience and support for my love and work with this art.

~ Julie Cisler

Thank you to Julie Cisler for her design and layout of this book. Her insights and artful expressions, book expertise, and Taiji ability, makes all my books works of art and great treasures. I couldn't do this without her!

Thank you to Margo Bock for compiling, editing, and the Willow #2 artwork. She caught so many edits, offered great ideas, and kept us on track!

Thank you to Dan Dale for photo and image quality control, and for shooting my 2024 photos.

Thank you to Rose Davis for the Willow #1 photos.

Thank you to all the contributors for your heartfelt and insightful recollections, photos, and remembrances.

Thank you to Joanne and Phil Von Blon for believing in me and supporting my teaching and my art.

Thank you to Master T.T. Liang for setting me on this path, with this art, in this beautiful land of lakes, the state of Minnesota.

Last but never least, I would like to thank all my students for forty years of magical, productive, and inspiring Taiji classes. I bow to the ground...

~ Ray Hayward

The Seventh Generation Speaks

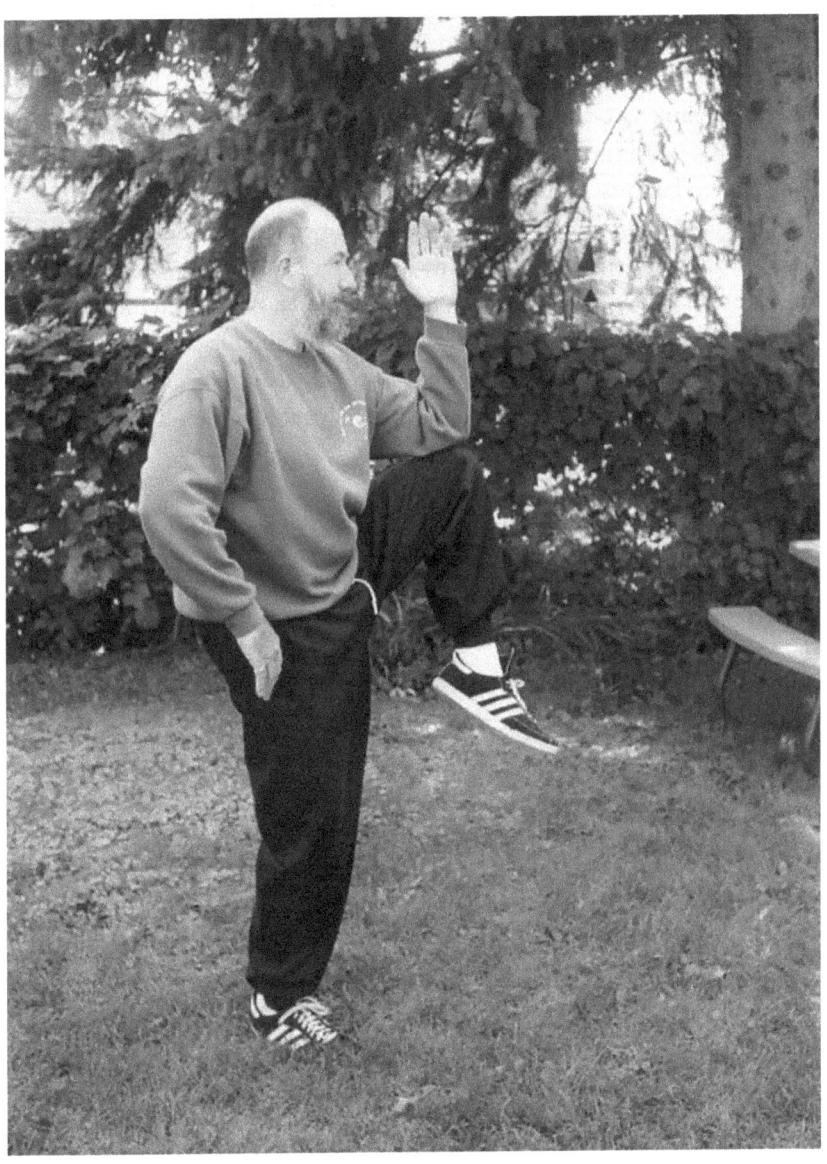

Intro by Margo Bock

In the following pages, we, the students of Ray Hayward, a 6th-generation Yang Style Taiji lineage holder, have put into words the genuinely felt impact of our beloved Taiji teacher as he marks four decades of enlightenment and guidance based in Minnesota. Through the voices of his dedicated students, we delve into the transformative journey sculpted by his knowledge, patience, and deep experience as a teaching martial artist. Each testimonial illuminates the profound ways in which our teacher has imparted the inner workings of Yang Style Taiji as handed down from Master T.T. Liang, Grandmaster Wailun Choi, Master Paul Gallagher, Dr Leung Kay-chi, and others; additionally, this collection chronicles how Sifu Ray has nurtured an interactive learning environment for personal growth and self-discovery in people of many backgrounds through instruction in mediation, Qigong, martial arts weapons, Xingyi, Bagua and more. Join with us by reading personal narratives on his inspired legacy in Minnesota while we honor the countless lives he has touched and the enduring spirit of discovery, health and relaxation he has cultivated within our Taiji circle.

Daniel Dale

I have been exceedingly lucky to have met Master Ray Hayward and even more lucky to study with him and be allowed to benefit from his life's work, his many teachers and his decades of teaching. I've had a number of teachers in a number of styles and truly have seen the worst and some pretty good ones. I have been a long time follower of Master Liang and his 150 posture Yang style form since the mid seventies and was fortunate to meet and show how his writings had put me on this life long roller coaster or better yet say adventure.

Even before meeting Sifu Hayward I had been reading his book "Lessons With Master Liang" I had also been viewing his work online like the small space series of lessons on Patreon. I soon was attending Sifu's classes and I started perceived a notion that maybe to him these arts may not be some antique form of exercise or self defense handed down by the ancients, but also a living art. A work of art that with the deep understanding, knowledge and refinement of each master's hand we see this amazing treasure live and evolve. Master Hayward is one of those skilled artists.

As an example: imagine the artist who buys the paint, the canvas and makes a wonderful work of art. But then realize the greatest artists reflect on and study the canvas, the paint even glue pondering the limitations in the how and why of how it is used. That's the difference in a Master Artist, and he may not be a painter but this is exactly the level and depth and great insight I see with Master Hayward. Even if he was not my teacher I would surely still most humbly bow from the waist to him. But at last I am the lucky one.

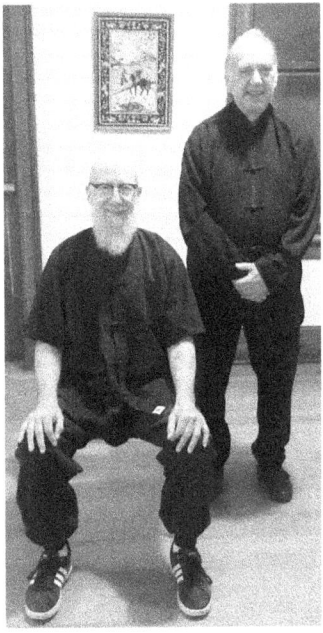

Season Of Blooming Flowers In The Year of the Wood Dragon

Really Bad Dan

Margo Bock

In Honor of Sifu Ray's 40th Anniversary in Minnesota: a poem about my experience as his student

Many evening & day classes seeded my
Inner development
Never compromising taiji principles
Notebooks mark my journey
Ever continuous the flow
Such is the way Sifu Ray teaches
Over everything else
Training for growth; physical and spiritual
Any and every day of the year

Margo Zi Yan
7th Generation Yang Style Disciple
2024

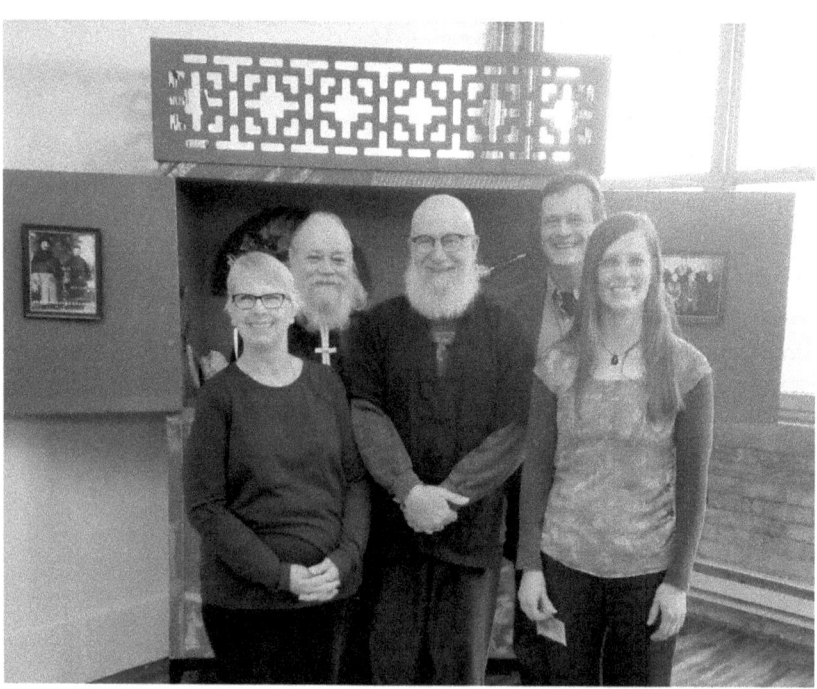

Jerry DeWees

Sifu Ray is very skillful and very good at passing on what he has learned over many years of dedicated study. He is kind, caring, patient, understanding, and always has words of encouragement when I'm having trouble figuring something out. Basically, he's everything I look for in an instructor. I consider myself extremely fortunate to be able to study Taiji with him and hope to do so for many years to come. (He's fun to hang out with outside the studio, too!)

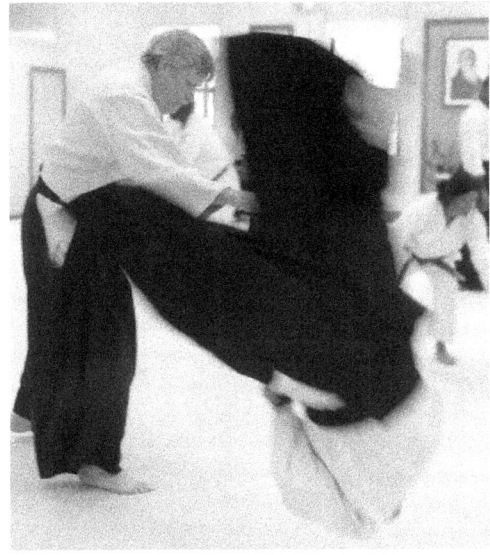

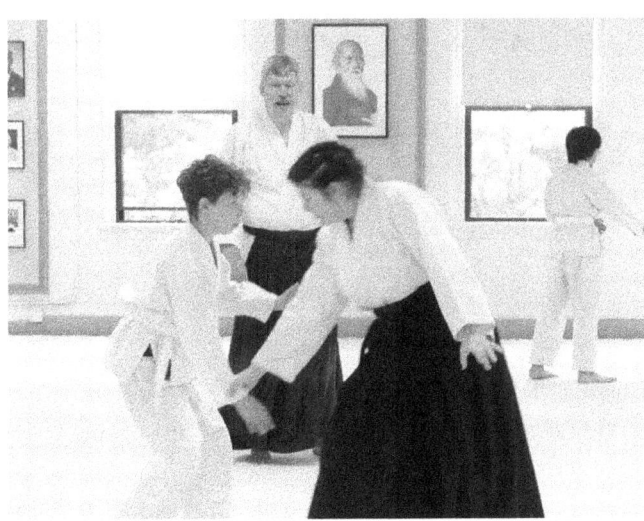

Matthew Barrett

I thought I had a million pictures of you. Turns out those pictures are mostly in my memories. The pictures in my mind have sensations associated with them. My first struggles at the form, watching how calmly and surely you did the form, the feeling of comfort and being in the right place.

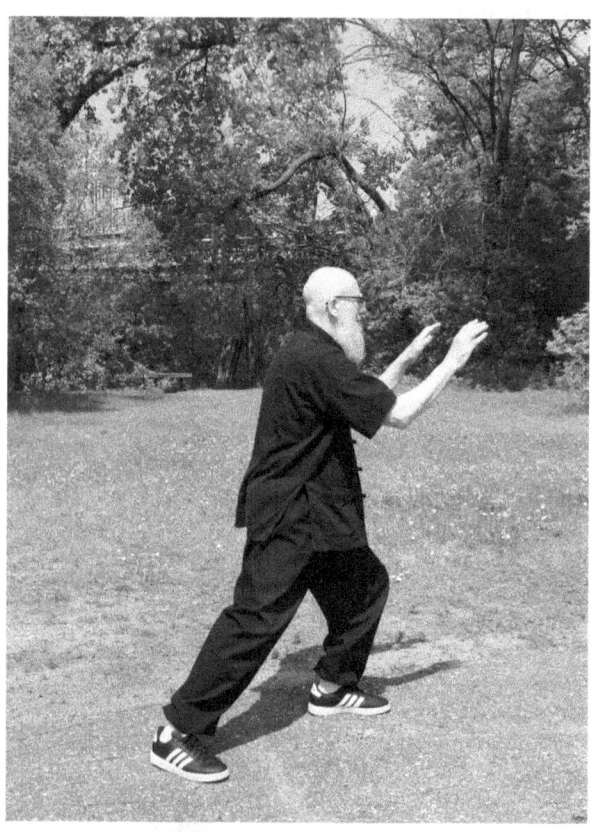

The first time I saw a slight wobble in your form. I thought, OMG, he is actually a human being :) The feeling that you were not upset, deterred, thrown off by what happened, you simply kept going with the same sense of confidence. It's a state that I strive to be in.

I know the cadence of your teaching. The gentle and not as gentle reminders. The 100 million ideas that you share. The slow progress of my learning. Taking the words, the example, the corrections, the praise, and making the form my own. My favorite picture of you is simply sharing space and time with you.

Paul Ittner

My journey studying taiji with Sifu Ray Hayward began in 2012 upon returning from visiting my daughter in Beijing, China. I was so inspired by watching all the Chinese people practicing taiji in the parks and temples, that I promised myself I would continue my own study in Minneapolis. I had practiced taiji in the 80's and 90's with a community education class and various other schools, but I stopped for 9 years.

When I met Sifu Ray at Twin Cities Tai Chi Chuan, I knew I had found a masterful and inspiring teacher. Sifu Ray is a patient, detailed, fun and knowledgeable instructor. Since Ray has been practicing and teaching martial arts for most of his life, and has studied with Master T.T. Liang, Grandmaster Wai-lun Choi, Grandmaster Gin Foon Mark, Dr. Leung Kay-chi, and many other martial artists, I realized I had opened the door to learn from a true master.

Now, I am learning and practicing an awe-inspiring warm-up and stretching routine, standing meditations, several chi kung forms, and complete taiji, bagua, and xingyi systems, including weapons forms. Sifu Ray also teaches the applications with these forms, and push hands practices. The philosophical, spiritual, health, and martial arts aspects are all part of these teachings. Sifu Ray seems to attract serious, diverse, and interesting classmates to his school. I really look forward to each and every class and practicing what I've learned at home. Practicing taiji and related

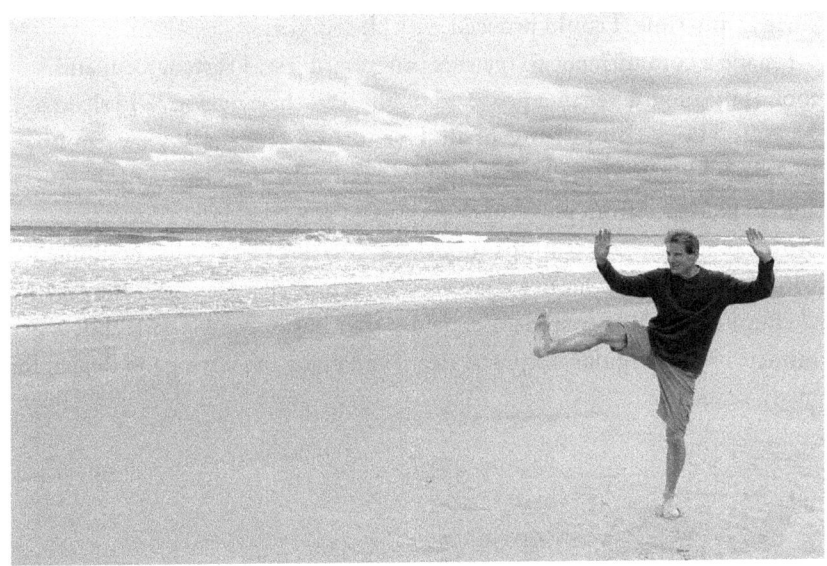

arts almost everyday is enhancing every aspect of my life. Taiji for me is truly meditation in motion.

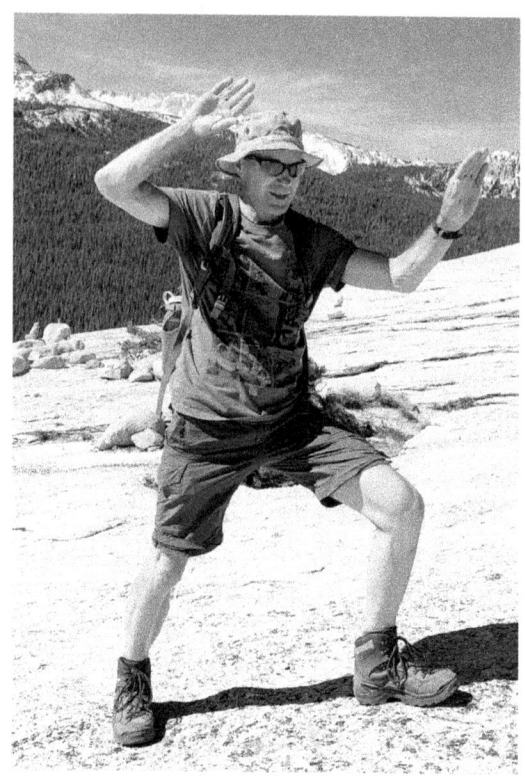

My career as a chef for 45 years was very mentally and physically demanding. In 2014, I developed some lower back problems (ruptured discs, stenosis, spondylolisthesis, and arthritis) and could barely walk. I was a candidate for triple back fusion surgery. I talked to Sifu Ray about this dilemma. Sifu suggested I use the taiji stretching and warm-ups, standing meditation, physical therapy, and time before proceeding with the surgery. This seemed wise, since at any time, I could proceed with the surgery.

I made a commitment to try this program. First, I rested, iced, and took Ibuprofen. I began a program of physical therapy with Physicians Neck and Back Clinic. Most of all, I went through Sifu Ray's warm-ups and stretching at least twice a day. Gradually, the pain lessened. I was able to graduate from physical therapy, and stop the daily Ibuprofen. Now I practice the warm-ups first thing EVERYDAY! That combined with the taiji long form has enabled me to enjoy life without 3 metal chunks in my lower spine! I consider that not only a blessing, but a miracle. With regular Taiji practice, I can enjoy life with good health for many years.

Wanda Koehler

My guess is that most of Master Ray Hayward's long-time students started their Tai Chi journey with him from their very introduction to the art.

My path, however, was less direct. My first lessons in Master T. T. Liang's Tai Chi Ch'uan Long Form was from someone who had no known affiliation with Sifu Ray. Subsequently, my learning continued with students of Sifu Ray. While each of them had different presentation styles, they all said the same thing regarding the techniques and principles of Tai Chi that they were learning from their teacher, Master Hayward.

The first time I met Sifu Ray was at a Chinese New Year Demonstration. I was mesmerized and in awe. How could I learn some of those forms? The answer came a few years later when Sifu began teaching at Carleton College. Later, I had the opportunity to go to Minneapolis to Mindful Motion Academy and take many classes. My learning level went up exponentially. It was wonderful to learn from Sifu Ray. While I'm a little tongue tied around my teacher, my plan was to learn everything possible. I listened intently to Sifu, took copious notes and learned from listening to his answers to other student's questions.

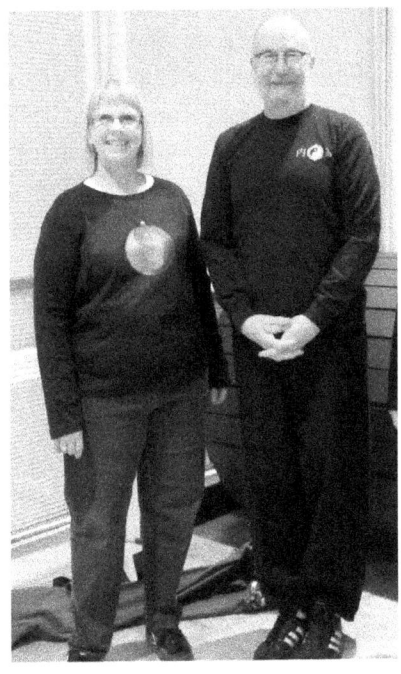

Eventually at Sifu's request, I began teaching the Tai Chi class through the Carleton College Rec Center. That ended with the pandemic. Late in the summer of 2020 with social distancing in mind, I taught classes in a local park. Currently, I teach a private lesson in my home. None of these opportunities would have happened without learning from a great teacher like Sifu Ray.

Tai Chi Ch'uan has been truly a joy for me. And having the privilege of learning from a teacher with the level of skill and knowledge that Master Ray Hayward possesses, is a treasured gift in my life.

John Feeley

"Find your teacher and good things will arise."

I started my Martial Arts journey beginning with Tae Kwon Do. The first Karate dojo I looked at was 7 minutes from my house, very convenient. I studied there for many years and progressed through all the skilled belt levels earning a black belt, became proficient at sparring, and eventually taught at the dojo. My Tae Kwon Do journey came to an end when I decided to explore a different style of martial arts, as I desired to learn more about the internal sense of balance and energy flow.

My exploration led me to T'ai-Chi Ch'uan. As I searched for a teacher, I found myself reflecting on how fortunate I was to have had the caliber of teachers I did in Tae Kwon Do. Eventually, I came across a teacher who was located close by. I learned, practiced, and taught for several years. During that time, I also ventured out to observe and joined in with other folks practicing at parks in my community, read many Tai Chi books, and bought DVDs, all in my search and craving to gain deeper knowledge. I came to realize there was much more to learn about this simple appearing yet intricate art. During one of my visits to a martial arts store, I purchased a book entitled Lessons With Master Liang. The author, Ray Hayward, was a T'ai-Chi instructor who was within driving distance to me, and I started to study with him.

The drive to and from my home to attend classes was much longer than I had initially anticipated, and the classes went much later at night. I vividly recall the winter nights, driving home from class late at night on the ice-glazed, dark county roads in subzero temperatures questioning, Is this all worth the effort?

Several years later I passed through a formal ceremony and ritual to be received and initiated as an inner-door student, the personal disciple (To-Di) of Sifu Ray Hayward, and a 7th Generation lineage holder in Yang-Style T'ai-Chi Ch'uan.

Was it all worth the effort? Yes! I continue my studies with Sifu Ray, and I am actively passing on the knowledge I have gained from him to my own students, offering them the good fortune of discovering my teacher.

"Find your teacher and good things will arise."
~ John Feely
Inner-door student of Sifu Ray Hayward

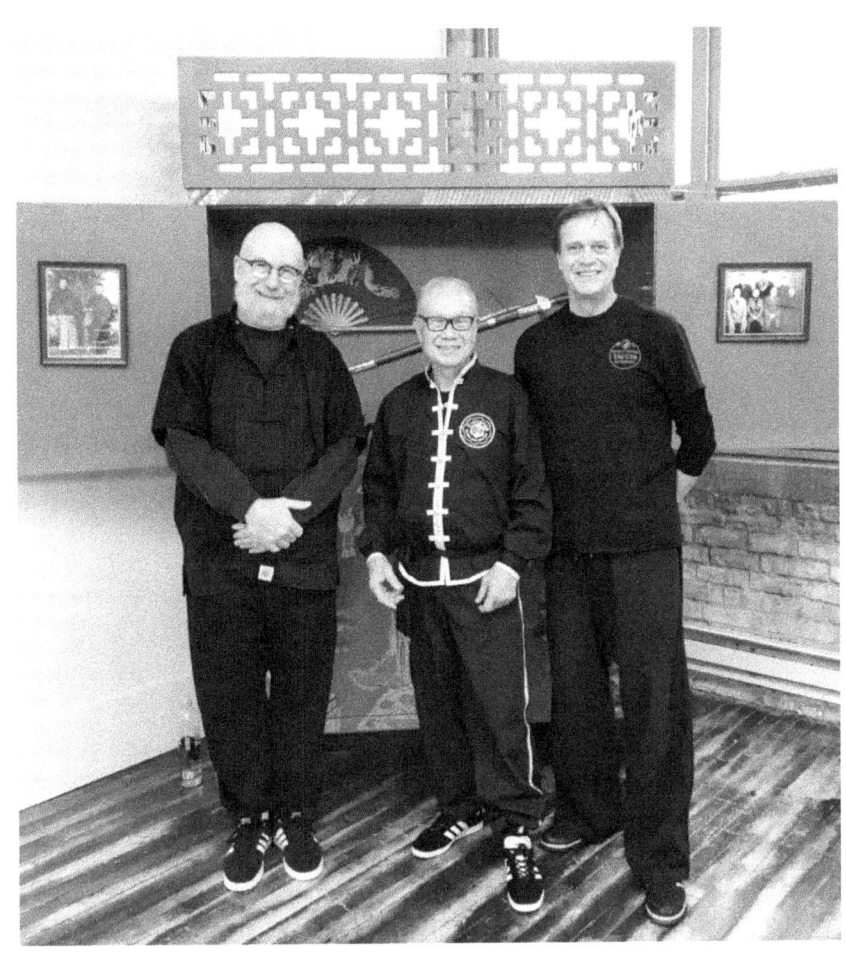

Michelle Ashmun

Tell me, what is it you plan to do with your one wild and precious life?
~ Mary Oliver

I will study with Sifu Ray, that is what I will do. Why? Because it feeds my wildness in healthy ways and delivers innumerable precious returns for my time and energy. (While the quote says wild and precious, I don't believe that I can separate them, so they intertwine and meld into a wild preciousness or precious wildness). I get to study with a teacher who has both a deep and broad knowledge that he has gained from studying and "eating bitter" with masters of direct lineages. He treasures his teachers and what he's learned from them and shares this legitimate, precious, hard-earned knowledge with me. This is rare, beautiful knowledge that you can't just get from a book. Having this knowledge fills me with gratitude and fulfills my need to have an interesting, adventurous life of unique experiences, wisdom, inspiration, and growth. It makes me grateful to be alive and to have a body, so that I can have these experiences.

And what an adventure, as I know Sifu Ray can supply me with an endless potential for learning and further inspiration. Sifu Ray readily shares his knowledge and directs me to books and resources on subjects I'm interested in so I can gain greater depth of knowledge. In addition to martial arts, I have opportunities to learn about Taoist philosophy and spirituality, Chinese history and culture, energy, meditation, Chinese medicine, and various health topics. Then there's the studies about the martial arts, such as style and lineage history, origin and evolution of forms, the Classics and related literature, theory, and strategy. This means I get to understand at a deeper level, because I can learn the "why," not just the "how." Furthermore, many of these topics become multifaceted metaphors for life lessons to inspire ways of life and pursuit of character strengths such as discipline, patience, and wisdom. To me, martial arts are a physical representation of character strengths and present innumerable opportunities to embody them. They teach me to navigate life wisely and become a better person so I can healthily embrace this wild, precious life of mine.

And then there's studying the martial arts themselves with Sifu Ray. I have the chance to learn the complete Tai Chi system, in addition to other martial arts that are not commonly taught, like Pa Kua, Hsing I, and Praying Mantis. I get to learn the form and drills, receive detailed and precise corrections, and learn the applications. Sometimes I pause to appreciate how it feels deliciously wild that I swing swords as part of my normal daily life. Anyways, I also get to witness and absorb Sifu Ray's modifications and innovations within these martial arts. I appreciate these changes as provides transparency by explaining his rationale for the modifications. I enjoy seeing how Sifu Ray demonstrates the "art" in martial arts. I also trust his judgment, as I know it is based on his own earnest studies and diligent practice.

There's another aspect of Sifu Ray's judgment that has contributed to my learning and growth, and that is his vision of me and my potential. I don't know what he sees in me, as I just show up to class and do my thing. But for whatever reason, he has recruited me to roles in performances and demonstrations and allowed me to work with his advanced students. While I was both honored and intimidated, I decided to have faith in his vision and determined to honor him by doing my best to live up to it. I had the opportunity to perform a sword versus fan form Sifu Ray created, perform an elbows-focused Praying Mantis 2-person form, and be a part of the Lion Dance team. Such wild, precious adventures! Ones that I will cherish always. In this way, Sifu Ray has given me opportunities to fulfill my potential and see my own bravery, determination, and strength that I didn't know I had.

I am profoundly grateful that Sifu Ray gave me opportunities to learn and do things that are deeply meaningful and I am proud of. A great way to make use of my wild and precious life.

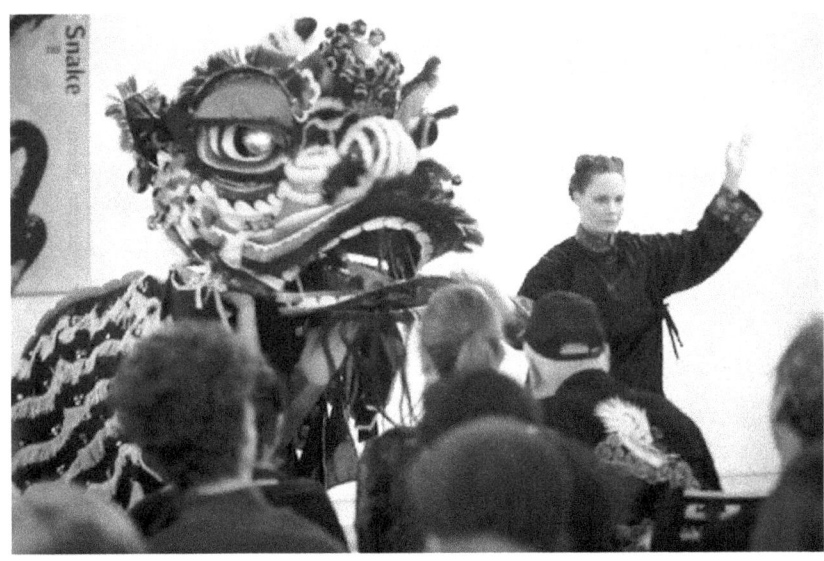

Robert Wozniak

There was a time when I left the studio because I felt I needed to get something from the harder, more external arts I had practiced before I met Sifu. Perhaps something wild still in me I needed to come to terms with. During this time I distinctly remember how much Sifu's teaching informed my external arts practice. Ultimately it informed me that Tai Chi was a much better fit for me, to put it mildly. So after a few years, and a few injuries, and a few wrong turns, I returned to Tai Chi and to Sifu. Not long after my return Sifu asked me to help a fellow student with the first few postures in the first section of the long form. I had been away for years, I thought this was going to be more of a hard lesson for me and a let down for my fellow student than anything else. But I was surprised by how much I remembered than I may have forgotten. I really helped this student! Helped me too. I realized that a great teacher can teach you more than you think you're learning.

40 years in MN, wow. Had I known 40 years ago what I know today, I'd be celebrating my 40th year practicing Tai Chi, in MN, with Sifu. So here's to the next 40!

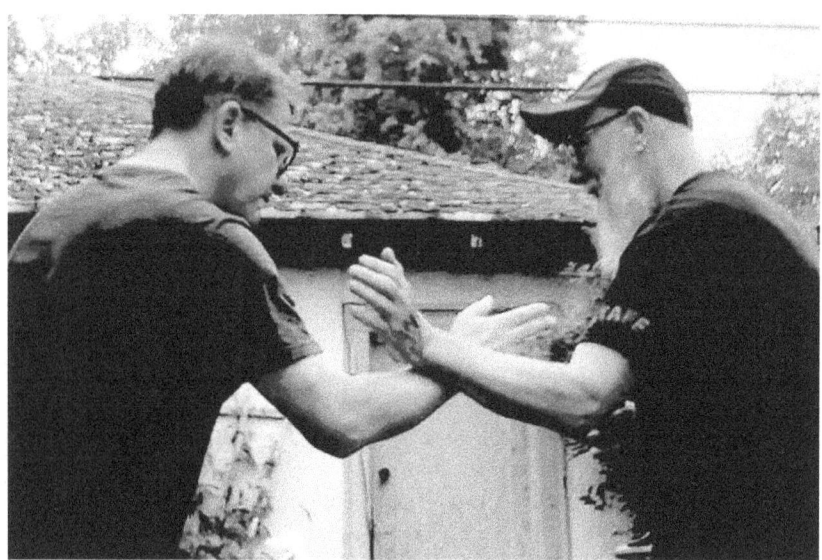

John Stitely

At first I take up T'ai Chi as a hobby,
Gradually I become addicted to it,
Finally I can no longer get rid of it.
I must keep on practicing for my whole life-
It is the only way to preserve health.
The more I practice, the more I want to learn
from teachers and books.
The more I learn, the less I feel I know.
The theory and philosophy of T'ai Chi is so
profound and abstruse!
I must continue studying forever and ever . . .
   ~ T. T. Liang

I began studying martial arts in about 1973. and continued for about 10 years, which is a saga for another time. I got quite strong in the process and learned some fundamental techniques. I thought I knew a lot, and when my teacher moved far enough away that I could no see him regularly, I took over his school and later opened my own school. In 1984, I closed the school and my family business and made the decision to go to Law School. This functionally terminated my martial arts practice until 2002, when I moved to Minnesota to be with a wonderful woman.

Neva was at that time taking introductory classes with a student of Twin Cities Tai Chi so I went along. It took me only a couple of lessons to start to remember what I had loved. In a few months the student terminated his class and introduced us to Sifu Hayward. Pretty soon I was coming to nearly every class I was eligible for. I underwent the education of both how little I knew but also how much I had wrong. Humbling but also exciting. I was continually being challenged to change in small and large ways to be better.

I have found my study with Sifu Hayward to be exciting. He teaches openly and even simple questions produce answers from a deep understanding that not only give the answer for the moment but sets the stage for future learning. Each element is later learned to have a deeper understanding, no matter how many times it is taught. Some of us students have used the phrase of "like drinking from a fire hose" to describe this experience. I say this knowing he hates the comment, but it is not meant as teaching so overwhelmingly as to leave us confused. He is a careful and detailed teacher, but he also consistently shows a glimpse to what we have yet to accomplish. It is both inspirational and aspirational rather than smothering.

I have over the years before and after beginning Tai Chi Chuan with Sifu Hayward, had contact with accomplished martial artists, taken seminars and the like. I have learned that the accomplishment of great skill and the ability to be a great teacher are not correlated. Master Hayward excels at a technical level that I cannot distinguish from those who he tells me are above him. He is also one of the best teachers I have ever seen. He is a master of both martial arts and the art of teaching. I am grateful to be his student.

After sixteen years of study I requested and was accepted as his disciple, and with it have accepted the duty to try and pass what I have been given. As a disciple of Sifu Hayward, I hold the lineage, at least in part, of those who are listed below. I, frankly, am barely qualified to mop the flour on which these people have practised, but Sifu Hayward has been supportive in my teaching and has proven to me that it is a path to deepening my understanding. He has also bestowed on me the honour of being one of the keepers of the Archives where he seeks to preserve what he knows so that these skills will not be easily lost. As part of this I have composed a Summary of this martial arts lineage.

Lineage, that is the list of who your instructors were and who their teachers were, etc. is a topic that usually makes Westerner's eyes glaze over much like reading the "begats" in Genesis. At one level it does not matter. It does not prove skill. It does not guarantee knowledge or understanding. For it offers some verification of the authenticity of what they have to offer.

Lineage is the short hand record of literally centuries of study, practice, experimentation, and understanding of martial concepts which have been passed to give the very best each teacher has learned to his descendants in the arts. Having the book does not mean you have understood it. It does not mean that you have it made part of your body, which is a significant part of what we mean when we say "master". It reminds us of the extraordinary accomplishments that gave us what we have and insofar as we learn them at least the "book" of their efforts is still "in print".

Sifu Ray Hayward began his health maintenance and Martial Arts training in 1973, studying Kenpo Karate and Jiu-Jitsu. In 1977, Ray met and began study with Master Tung Tsai (T. T.) Liang in Boston. Ray learned the complete Yang Style T'ai-Chi Ch'uan system from Master Liang, as well as Praying Mantis, Ch'i-Kung, Taoist Meditation, Ch'in-Na, Wu Dang Sword and various weapons. In 1984, Ray moved to Minnesota to continue studying with Master Liang. In 1988, Ray Hayward passed through a formal ceremony to become an inner-door disciple of Master Tung Tsai Liang. He also studied with Master William Chen privately for several years and hosted a seminar with him in Minnesota He also studied briefly with B. P. Chan and then studied with Chan's teacher , Dr. Leung Kay-chi, a renowned teacher and master. Ray Hayward had been given a formal introduction by Master Liang and from Dr. Leung he learned much, including but not limited to further instruction in Yang Style Taiji, Chen Style Taiji, Northern Shaolin, Yin style Bagua, and Xingi,

He studied Wu Style Tai Chi with Dr, Wen Zee (Cardiologist and Tai Chi Master whose teacher for several decades was the renown grandmaster Ma Yueh Liang, son-in-law of the founder of the Wu family style)

He was accepted as a disciple by Gin Foon Mark, Grandmaster of Jook Lum Southern Praying Mantis, and co-authored a book on that style describing the essential principles of that system. Sifu Hayward also learned Eagle Claw and Seven Star Praying Mantis from Lo Man-Biu.

For more than the last 20 years, Sifu Hayward has studied with the peerless Grand Master of Liu Ho Ba Fa, Wai-Lun Choi who taught him Xingi, Jiang Style Bagua, Taijiquan, Liu Ho Ba Fa and Yiquan.

It takes years of dedication to learn this body of knowledge. This is a level of study that is easily equivalent to several PhDs. Those that have this level of excellence are diminishing rapidly. Those who are willing to do this were never large in number and modernity is making it increasingly rare. We are fortunate to have him and the opportunities he offers and the example he shows us. Thank you Sifu.

Your devoted Disciple, John Stitely

Rondi Atkin

Initially I think you want me to quantify what I have learned from you, but on reflection I believe you want me to describe the experience of learning Taiji with you: that is, alongside you, and the first thing I know is that the place you teach from now is not the place you stood twenty years ago when I first started learning with you. The verb "to learn" comes from the same root as "footprint" or "to track." In this way, learning Taiji with you has become its own kind of Dao.

To learn Taiji with you is to venture beyond Taiji for health and meditation and to study it as a martial art—not for the purpose of being martial but to reify its art, knowing that without the martial there would be no art, no sublime, because learning Taiji with you has taught me that all things—in life as well as Taiji—contain their opposite and to hold it all. To learn Taiji with you is to know its essential energy, its qi, and how to cultivate and conjure it (such as recently, when I, a short person, had to hoist myself out of a dumpster and knew that it was qi as much as strength that lifted me). To learn Taiji with you means understanding the mechanics of my body and how I move in it, learning to use full body motion—not only when I do the Taiji form or attack/defend doing Pushing Hands, but also when I walk down the street, open a door, or roll out a pie crust.

To learn Taiji with you is to remember "first in the mind, then in the body" although the skeptic in me rejects its truth until each time I actually try to imagine doing a challenging posture (like I did a little while ago with Step Back and Sweep with Leg, imagining my left leg smoothly circling, my arms extended, my toe sweeping my fingertips, and as I did it in my body—Voila!— the closest I've gotten to the kick in my mind, like learning magic). To learn Taiji with

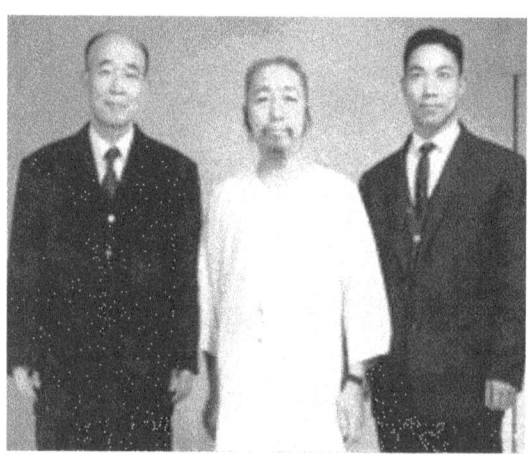

Hsu Fun Yuen (right), with Zheng Manqing and Liang Tungtsai (left).

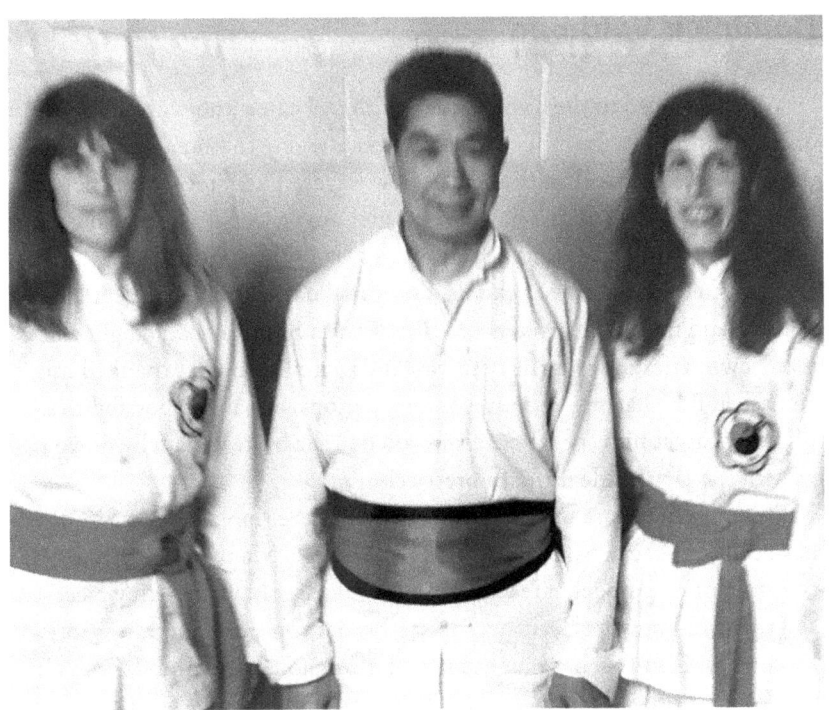

Hsu Fun Yuen (center), with Rondi Atkin (right), and Elizabeth Wenscott (left).

you is often to be frustrated, like how, because you too are always learning and refining our forms, you change the count or movement of a posture I have spent dozens of hours etching into my muscle memory only to have to sand away the old lines and etch in the new, but to learn Taiji with you is to walk this path of which the poet claims, "Traveler, your footprints / are the only road, nothing else." To learn Taiji with you is to learn from the many masters whose footprints you have followed, to track your devotion to your own training, to integrate the lessons culled from the breadth of your reading and observations of life, and to receive the gift of your teaching.

To learn Taiji with you, Sir, is to be brought deep into Taiji's heart, and even though what I achieve is light years from what is possible, the dive takes me higher, which may be why, no matter how low I might feel when I go to class, I leave feeling lifted–like being in love. To learn Taiji with you is to remember Master Liang's words: "Don't be concerned with being as good as Yang Lu-ch'an, just practice." To learn Taiji with you is to know there is no road–only footprints practicing in the sand.

Dominick Veldman

When I moved to the Twin Cities in 2000, I came knowing almost no one, and nothing about the town. I set about trying to find a Taiji school the way most people then did: the Yellow Pages. The internet was not then what it is now, and I didn't have a computer anyways. So as I'm cold calling school after school, looking for day classes (as I was working nights at the time) I asked one of those schools if they had day classes. The gentleman politely said no, but referred me to Sifu Ray, as Sifu Ray had taught this man's own wife, and was the best Taiji instructor in town. I thanked him and asked if he had any other recommendations, as backup possibilities. I'll never forget his reply; "I just told you he's the best. What else do you want?!" So that made my path pretty clear.

From my first class to my most recent, I've never looked back. Sifu Ray has been a most generous waterfall of knowledge. Many teachers go by the grain of rice model of teaching, where you are shown one tiny piece at a time, and must perfect that before they let you learn anything more. By contrast Sifu Ray has taught by the buffet model. He would always let you fill your proverbial plate, and it's your fault if you leave with mental digestive issues.

Some years ago, a handful of other students and I decided to try our hands at an open martial arts tournament in Madison. I opted to compete in Taiji weapons, Traditional Kung fu weapons, and Internal open hand forms. When I arrived, they also sought more participants for the Pushing Hands competition, so I thought "Sure!, sounds fun."

First came the Taiji Weapons. I came to do Taiji Sword. As part of the demonstration process, they inspect the weapons, to make sure they are sturdy, and won't break mid form and hit a judge. Well, I had brought my Arms and Armor prototype of Sifu's antique sword. So needless to say the Judge was surprised I'd brought an Actual Sword, instead of a wiggly wushu thing. I think he wanted to take it home himself.

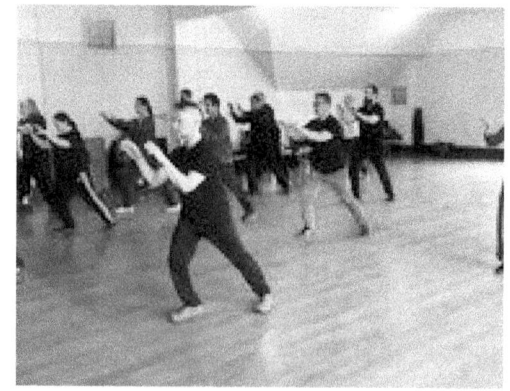

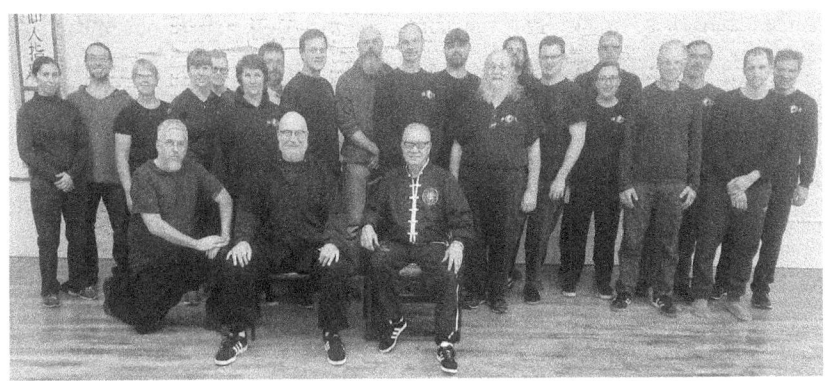

    I performed my form keeping in mind what Sifu Ray had related from Master Liang, "Practice as if it is a performance, and perform as if it were a practice." Everyone disappeared, and it was me and my form. In the end I recieved 1st place, and as the judges were giving their compliments and critiques, they asked me why my eyes tracked with the sword tip to so intensely. I told him what Sifu had taught us, that it helps us to extend our chi, or our awareness all the way through the weapon, helping to make it an extension of ourselves, and that it keeps us mindful of our surroundings, and where our opponent would be. He seemed surprised that I had a full explanation, but I'd just learned to take for granted that every inch of our practice has purpose. One of the other students there commented "I think I'd get motion sick trying that…"

    For the Wushu weapon, I performed 9 Section Whip. They again tested my weapon (it's like they didn't know me or something) I was fortunate and again got 1st.

    For the Chinese internal style I performed Xingyi 5 Elements Change form. I came in 2nd to a woman visiting from China, performing a Baji form. It was cool to see an internal style I'd had no previous exposure to. She approached me before the demonstrations, and said, "You do internal styles, don't you," I said, that I do, but asked what the give away was. She told me "It's your shoulders. All these hard style guys are sticking their chests out, but your shoulders are soft and relaxed." it was probably the highest compliment I got that day.

    At the end of the day was the Pushing Hands competition. I decided to try to approach it like practice. I did everything I could to just be as soft and yielding as I could, and to let them get stiff and tense. And it worked. A few of the competitors were obviously on the more beginner side, and rather than be a rude bully I was gentle about nudging them out of their stance. One older gentleman was a downright joy to work with. It was really like playing. Both of us taking delight in the others skill. My fiercest competitor was a younger man about my age, who was quite aggressive and just stiff enough to work to my advantage. The skill that the judges Pointed out in their final comments that got me through the most was how, instead of resisting or fighting I would drop my weight and root, turning or diffusing their push. Again the basics saw me through, and I took 1st.

The first lesson is so often the last lesson. Relax, sink, and breathe. And if you know where the best teacher is… what more are you looking for?
Sifu: Thank you for being my teacher, my mentor, my Master, and my friend. I look forward to to learning from you for all the years to come.

There is one more thing I wanted to add:
It is the most basic of teachers who teach what they were taught. The better teachers point to how they were taught, and how to teach it. Only the very best of teachers show you everything they know, tell you what they don't know, and teach you how to learn apart from them.
 I know this lineage of great teaching goes at least to Master Liang. Beyond teaching the Mastery of Yang style Taiji, this might be his greatest gift to us all. Where Master Liang didn't know, he didn't pretend to. Instead, he sent Sifu Ray forth, saying: "Go learn from him!" Giving us a generous wealth of styles, and forms outside of Master Liang's study to learn from, and teaching our own sifu how to learn away from his sifu.
 This is a unique and uncommon thing in almost any style, or art, and must not be discounted. Many teachers are jealous of what they know, and hold back the best for their favorites, if they show even them. It is the rarest and most gracious of Masters who pour out openly what they know, and point you beyond their own doors.
 This level of intellectual generosity does of course lead to the casting of pearls before swine. But this piglet is grateful to have at least touched on this string of pearls, and hopes to pass along some of it, someday. Thank you, ~Dominick Veldman

Michael Sauter

A Martial Father

I had the honor of studying and training under Sifu Ray Hayward for 13 years before leaving the Twin Cities. He taught me in the areas of Northern Praying Mantis, Southern Mantis, Bagua, Xing-Yi, and some other areas to varying degrees. I have since continued to work on consolidating and expanding my knowledge based off of his platform for now over 23 years. I don't think there are many teachers that can teach like Sifu can. From my experience he has continued to amaze me with his subtle nuance to any movement. Expanding ideas, and his pursuit to continual growth. Even if you don't study Tai Chi, his main art, you will find ways of leaching his persona into other arts. I often reflect on his mannerisms and just seeing a video or an image brings back the moments in class. In the old days he rarely was seen without a Studio sweat shirt even in the midwest humid summers. As a student you couldn't slack off to that, you tried as you might to control your energy... at least I did. There was always something to learn, like the way he could teach someone through another person has stuck with me into my management career. The many demos taught you how to perform in front of an audience. When I kept failing he called me out once and told me to do it again in front of a crowd. He always seemed to know what each person needed.

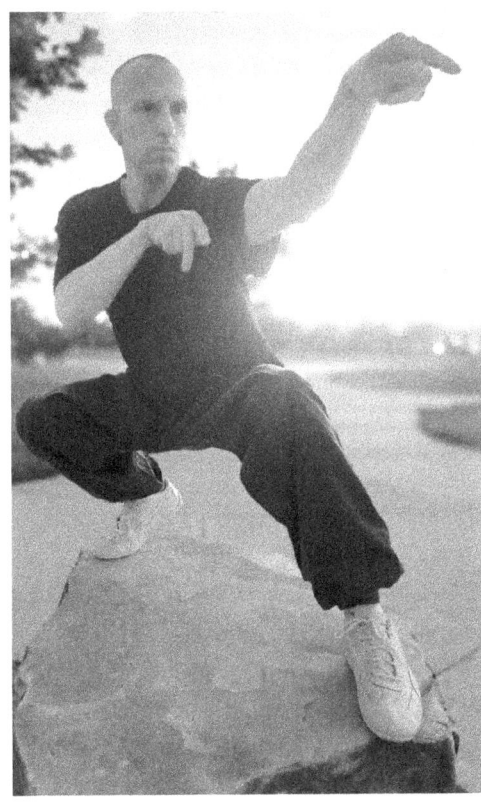

When I started training I was a bit younger and looking for something to have for my own. I used to watch kung fu movies with a friend, and practiced what we thought was sticky hands from Jet Li flicks. Its amazing to think in months I had more than I could ever imagine. Sifu didn't teach to sashes or ranks, though there were some depending on the style. He didn't teach tournament fighting or a bunch of parlor tricks. He always says that he gave out his art freely, like T.T. Liang would say. But you had to put in the work and time to find secrets. Many can take for granted what is taught to you in words or written in notes. Nowadays everything is watched online. His structured classes stick with me today as I continue my own training. The formula that keeps everything together. Warm-ups, Stances, punches, kicks, forms, partner work, sensitivity, and weapons. There are many forms most can learn if you put forth the effort. Again its consistent training over time that matters. Sifu has had a lot of long term students, many longer than me. I believe its because of his care for the arts that were past on to him by some great masters. I believe you can see elements of each one in his overall cadence, and the crook of his brow. Many stories live on through his telling.

Despite the school not normally having a tournament presence, I did go to a few to represent the school. This was a great time of advancement for me. And again Sifu never failed in having pointers in how I should approach sparring and forms presentations. He would say not to even bother on light sparring, it was pointless. Either do it or don't. So I entered the USKSF regional tournament in Madison, WI. The first year I went with my training partner Josh Lynch and entered the Lei Tai (full contact fighting), open hand forms, and weapons competitions. He and I grew a great bond during this time practicing everything we can imagine and taking a few blows along the way. I can recall nursing a broken rib and a deathly hit to the head during those days. But its all what it takes if your going to take it serious. I took home a few medals throughout the various areas I competed in on my trips. The last one being an International tournament in Baltimore, MD. I didn't fight in that one, but did a version of Damo Jian with tassel inspired by T.T. Liang who always liked tassels added to weapons.

I have also had the privilege to assist Sifu Ray in teaching Mantis curriculum back at the MN studio, held youth classes of my own, and have done some seminars. Now days I usually can be found out in the parks keeping up rotations. There were a lot of key moments in my training but two stand differently for development. I am by nature a creative person, I favor organic flow. I care about a motion sometimes more than the flat outcome. There can be passion and meaning in that. Like a perfect whisk of a pen stroke. I once was frustrated by rigidity in how we were practicing some forms. Sifu told me there are many ways of doing

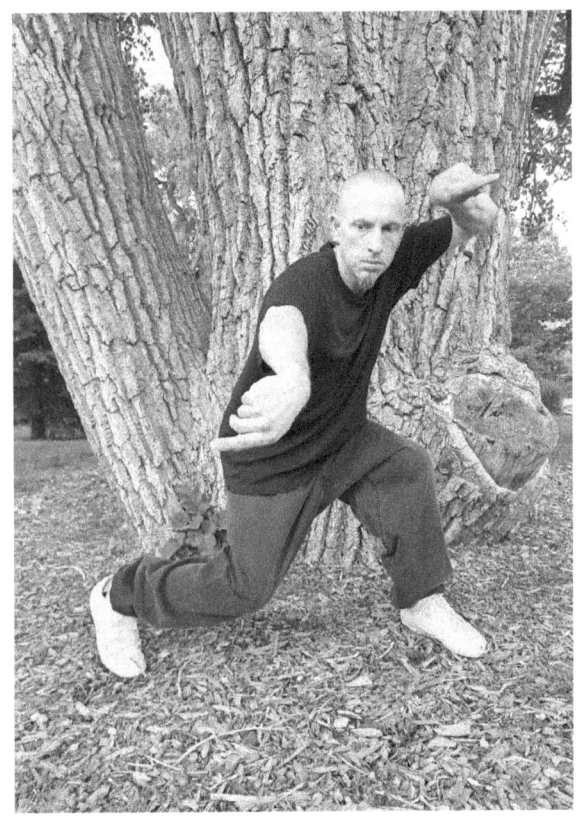

things. I don't recall the true words but basically find your own way. Another time Sifu said to me, you know that monkey foot work, swap them out for Xing-yi, see what you come up with. You didn't always know when or where he would suggest something. But you always knew he was watching. For me, these ideas sent me down a rabbit whole of training breaking down all my knowledge and putting them back together. When you train this way you need to understand each piece in order to know where your going. And how to come back. You look to limit wasted movements. You find alignments to create more with less. Apply fighting logic, and process all the energies, long, short, and segmented. Sifu Ray has truly left me with something I will be exploring for a long time to come. He has sent me to learn from others on our lineage, I find myself still process things through his methods. You can find people who can teach various things in this world but to me he is a martial father and represents his teachers before him!

Christopher Venaccio

Aerosmith once sang ""Cause Falling In Love Is So Hard On The Knees". But Tai Chi isn't, right? Keep your knees over your toes, make sure you can see the toes of your front foot past your knee, and let your structure support your weight. Pretty simple.

I've been fortunate to attend many workshops and retreats taught by Master Ray over the course of many years. Each has been filled with books' worth of information — details of the forms, history of the art, stories of the past masters, humor, comedy, music, and modifications.

Wait, modifications? You mean things change? Sometimes, yes, but always within principles and always for a specific reason or objective in the hands of a master.

It was in a workshop not so long ago (and not in that galaxy far, far away known as Minnesota) that Master Ray introduced a variant of Tai Chi Sabre. The big spins and big jumps were reduced or removed, much to my chagrin. It took me a long time to get those down. Gosh darn it, they should stay. Tai chi is about me, isn't it? I stay in the center and it moves in circles around me. Copernicus called to tell me I was wrong.

In one of the breaks between sessions, I was able to have a short conversation with Master Ray about the modifications.

"I'm saving knees, both my own and other's," he said. He quickly picked up on my "honestly, is it really that hard on your knees?" expression. "At your age," he continued, "you can still easily do those postures as they have been handed down, but talk to me when you are 50. Then again at 60. After an injury. Or when you are teaching people in their 60's. Or on a surface that is rough or sticky."

My Tai Chi forms are practiced on very forgiving surfaces 95% of the time - hardwood floors that are smooth or perhaps dusty (with shoes with very little grip), cut grass in parks, etc. It's easy to spin or land a jump on those without jarring your body. Rarely am I practicing forms on rocks, concrete, wet grass, or even sand. So infrequently in fact that I never gave the surface much thought because I always had a more optimal surface available.

As I have grown older in the art and have had students of wider age ranges and physical abilities in classes, I have found that having these variants in your back pocket is a key to longevity in the art, both in my own practice and in being able to teach others. Did I mention that masters give you gifts at the oddest times? Congratulations on your 40 years in Minnesota, Master Ray! ~Christopher Venaccio

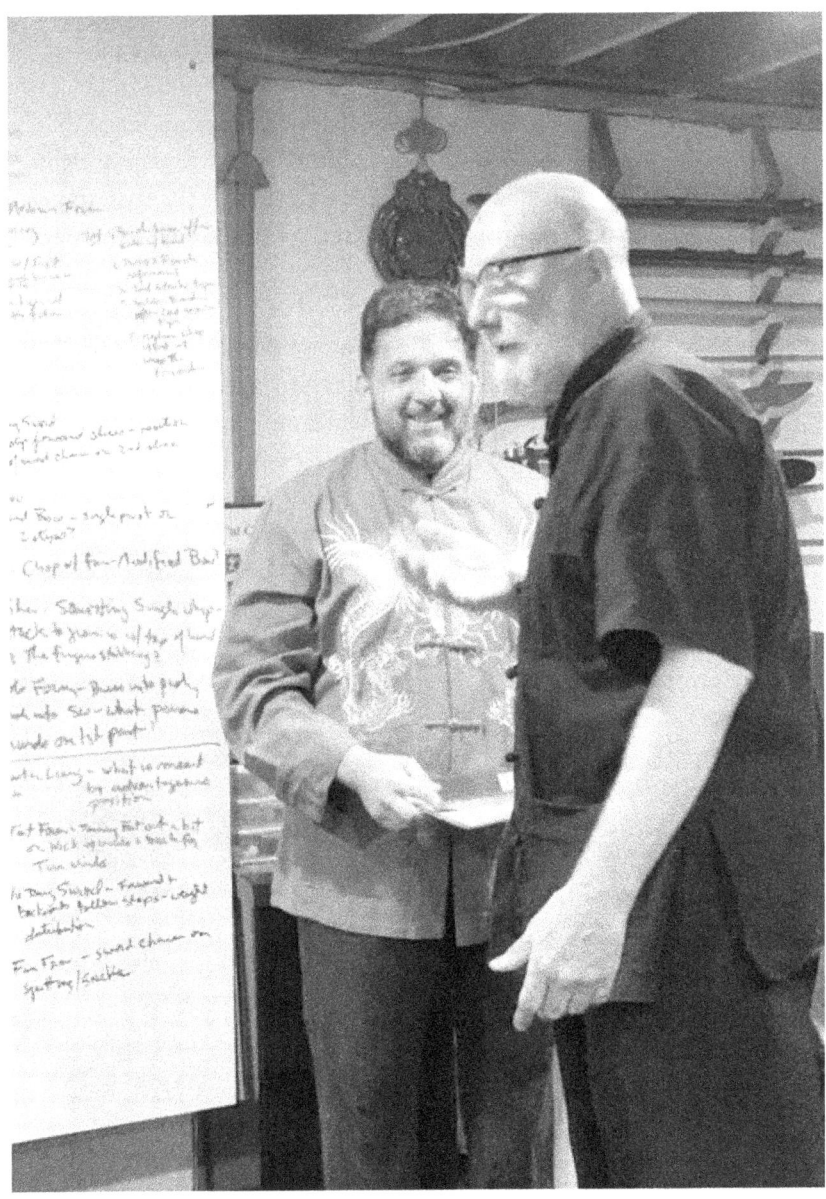

Karen Barton

The Altar Opening

I have been Sifu Ray's student for nearly twenty years. From retreats, to private lessons, to moments where he boosted my confidence, there are many anecdotes I could recount as meaningful. One of my favorite memories is of a beautiful sunny day in May 2022 when he opened my home altar.

I am fortunate enough to have a home dojo filled with equipment to support my physical health. My walls are adorned with weapons, weights, and mats. Of all the tools I have in that space, the altar is the most important piece of equipment. It serves to strengthen my connection to masters in our lineage old and new.

For the ceremony, a small group of classmates joined us in lighting incense and setting intentions for future practice. Sifu Ray gave a brief talk describing the altar as a "portal" to the old masters who have passed along to another plane and to others in our Tai Chi family who have altars in their homes. Every time I light incense before a practice session, I look into the eyes of the old masters on the black and white photos and ask for their assistance. Sometimes I need extra discipline to get through the forms I have on my schedule that day. Sometimes I need a boost of mental energy to stay focused. And sometimes I need a push simply to start the warmups. The masters never fail my requests. As the flame on the incense dims to an ember, I think of my classmates practicing in their homes and the collective alchemy of peaceful energy we create together. The portal works, every time.

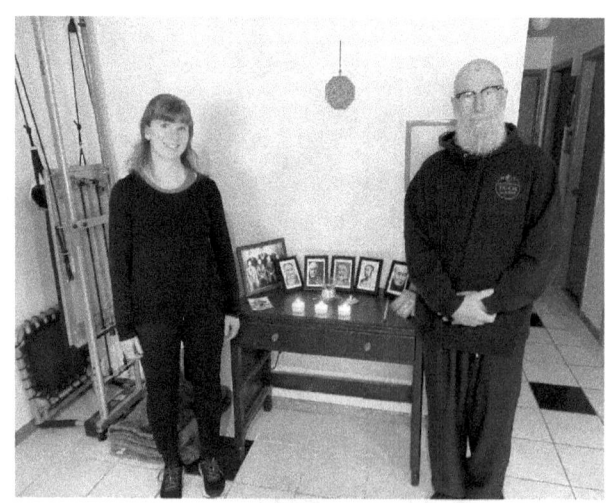

Sifu Ray and me directly after the ceremony.

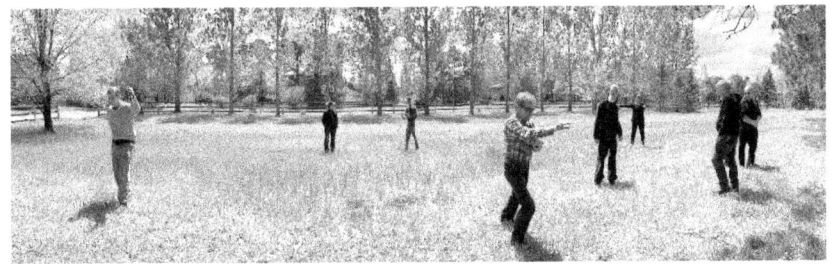

Everyone practicing forms they started.

After the ceremony, through the fog of incense smoke, Sifu did something I had never seen before and have not seen since. Each person in attendance was asked: what form do you want to start today? It had to be a new form, not something we had learned once and allowed to fade away. It had to be brand new. I chose the fan (which I subsequently took almost two years to learn and demonstrated for the 2024 Chinese New Year demo). Others settled on sword with tassel, daggers, and other empty handed forms.

Just as my altar opening was a new beginning for my spiritual journey, all in attendance were now invited to begin something new on their tai chi journeys. The group relocated from my basement dojo to my yard to begin learning. Sifu Ray rotated between us by showing each person a posture or two and then moving to the next person while we practiced what we had just learned. It was a beautiful day.

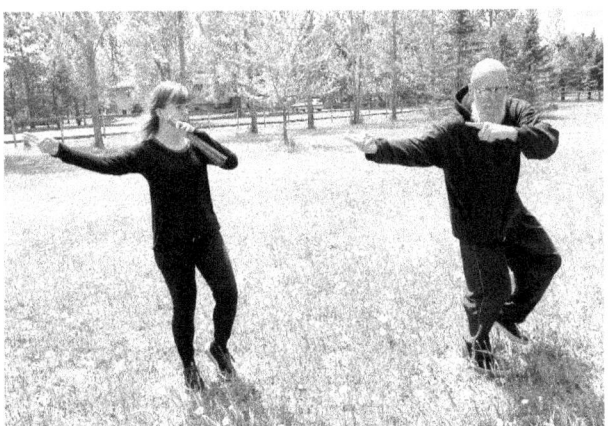

Me learning "the immortal guiding the road" - the second posture of the fan form.

Martin Ebelhardt

A Few Reflections on a Taiji Journey with Master Ray Hayward

I first met Master Ray Hayward in 2004 after a Doctor of Traditional Chinese Medicine recommended Taiji to help me heal after a serious knee injury. I remember fondly my first contact with the man who would become both my teacher and friend. His warmth and careful attention to what he was teaching, and to the progress of his students struck me. I had been around some very high-level martial arts masters in my life, and can say that not all give what they have to teach so freely. One of the many things I have always admired about Ray is that he gives you everything that's in his cup to give.

After the first few months of study watching him teach and guide, listening to his explanations of the postures, health benefits, history of Yang Taiji and of his lineage, it was apparent to me that I was in the presence of a highly skilled teacher, and I was pretty strongly grounded in my interest of continuing to study Taiji as his student. I continued to walk the path, grew to love Taiji and through the years built a daily practice. I loved going to the studio, looked forward to the drills, the camaraderie, and especially loved the blackboard lessons in which we went deep into everything. I recall him many times saying that the fundamentals, and basic principles were vital to learning and embodying the art at its deepest level.

As is common in life, life happens and as the years wore on I went through some major life changes including a divorce, a second marriage, becoming a parent. Life got busy! Although I continued to practice daily, my ability to make it to the studio became less and for several years I only made it to the studio occasionally, then eventually stopped going at all. I practiced at home, but not every day and kept it alive, but just barely.

After a few years of time away from the studio I started to do some private lessons with Ray, and began by letting him know that I felt bad about being away, citing my dismay about my busy life with work and kids, some chronic pain issues that were limiting my practice and about wishing I had more time to learn and study all that he had to offer, including Xingi, Bagua, and Li Ho Pa Fa. I also mentioned that I had fallen away from weapons practice and had only really been doing the empty hand form and a little sword, and some days just drilling individual postures and some standing meditation. You could say the wind was out of my Taiji sails and I was feeling very bad about it.

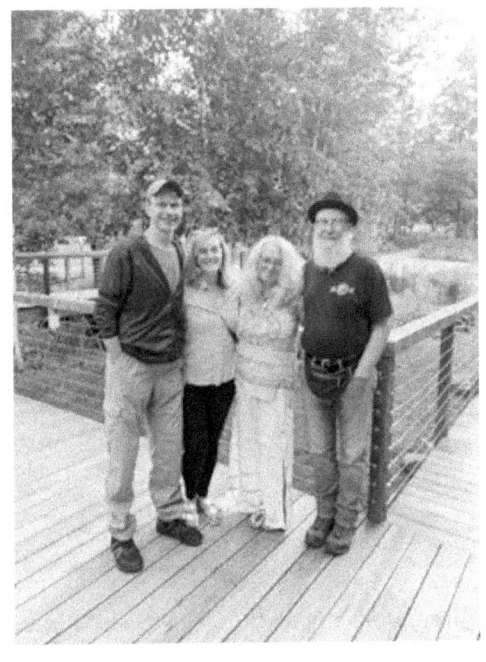

He could have just said don't worry or dismissed my concern, but instead he essentially breathed life back into what felt like a deflated balloon in my practice. He explained that it was not about how much you study or how many arts, nor did it matter if you have to step away or dial down your practice. He told me life gets busy, so you do what you must and keep up with it as best you can. When you have more time you do more, when you have less time you do less. He said, "Taiji is in you because you have already learned the forms from all the dedicated hours of training, so it will come back. Tailor your practice to your life, not your life to your practice."

He then shared with me that Master Zheng Manqing only practiced Taiji and only trained the Sword and no other weapons, and that he ascended to a very high level of skill. Then, started to teach small bits of Hsing Yi, and Bagua impressing upon me that I did not need to do the entire system. This is only one of the many lessons that really helped me along during difficult times in my life. There are so many more, and so many other moments on my Taiji journey that I treasure and will hold deep in my heart, in my soul and in my being for the rest of this journey.

In 2018 I began to pass along the art to others. I consider it a great honor and a responsibility I don't take lightly. I hope that I am able to provide even a small amount of the illumination for others, that he has provided and continues to provide for me.

Although I will always regard Ray with the utmost respect first and

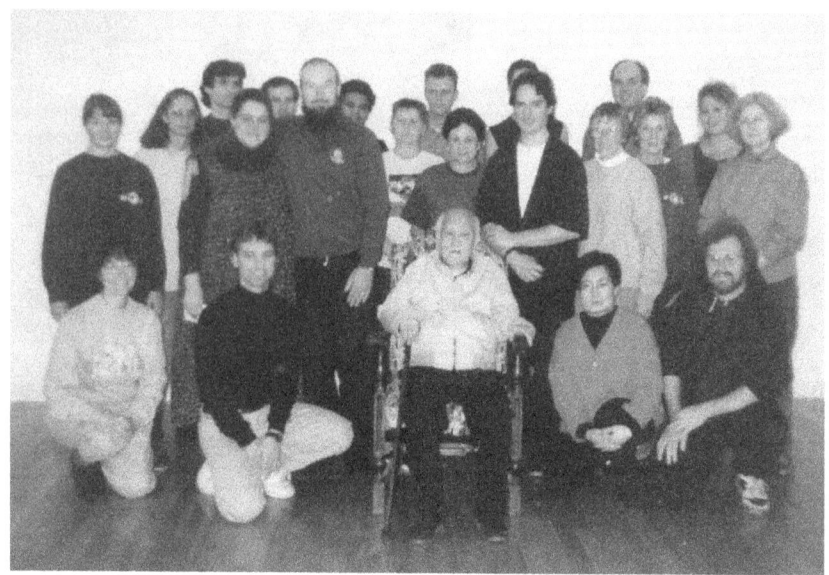

foremost as my teacher, he has also been such an important part of the fabric of my life as a mentor a guide, and especially as a friend. You will find very few people in this life who truly accept you for who you are, who love you without judgement, and who don't put you into some sort of a conceptual box with some expectations about who or how you should be. If you have the good fortune to be in his presence, then you know what I mean!

Happy 40th Taiji Anniversary Master Ray, my teacher and good friend!

Sharon Nyberg

When I first walked into the studio, I had carpal tunnel so severe that I couldn't straighten my fingers. I used a voice-activated computer at work. I needed both hands to lift a carton of milk. I had been to many doctors, the last of whom had me on 3,000 mg of aspirin a day. Nothing had worked. I finally said, "Enough!" and resigned myself to living with the condition. Then I heard about tai chi. I thought - "Why not? What have I got to lose?" One day during standing meditation, with my hands held in front of my chest, I saw flames shoot out of my fingertips. It was so startling and weird that I kept it to myself for a long time. But the more I practiced tai chi, the more I came to believe that those tongues of fire I saw in my mind's eye were the release of blocked energy from carpal tunnel. It's been about 30 years and my fingers are straight; my hands are strong and flexible. Tai chi helped my body heal itself, when nothing else did. I'm grateful you moved to Minnesota, Ray. Congratulations on a remarkable 40 years.

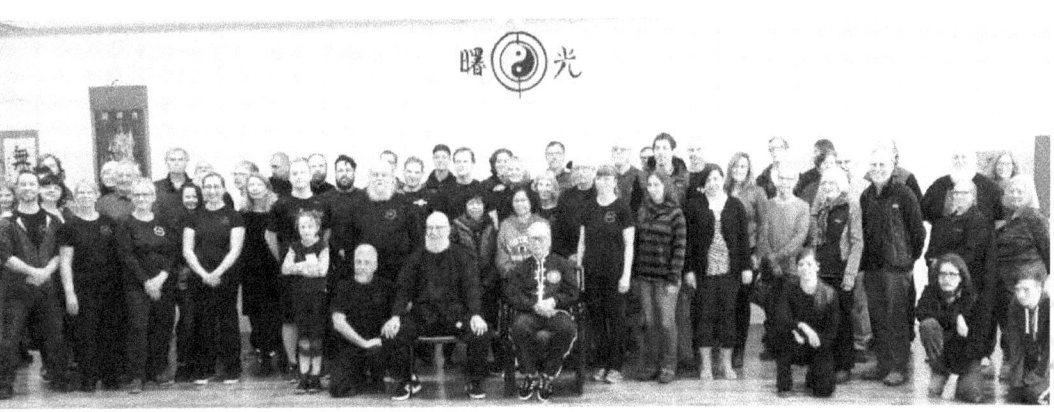

Michael Cain

Serendipity, Providence, and an Arc of Illumination

Growing up in the 1960s and 1970s, Eastern marital arts were all the rage. From Bruce Lee to "Kung Fu" (the series) to Chuck Norris, it seemed everyone was a fan, if not a budding practitioner. During my elementary school years, we lived in New Orleans, Louisiana. My dad was fortunate enough to be a student of a famous Karate instructor who was recently transplanted into the deep south from Japan. Other than brief glimpses of a kata or some technique being worked on, we rarely witnessed any demonstrations. Nevertheless, a seed had been planted.

In the Fall of 1978 I showed up as a freshman on the campus of Northeast Missouri State University with the idea that I could find a club, faculty member, or ROTC officer that might be offering some sort of martial arts instruction. Through the grapevine I was introduced to an older college student fresh out of the Coast Guard who happened to be leading a club. After the appropriate interviews and discussions, he suggested I join their "kung fu" class, which I was told, focused on the softer, more internal aspects of the arts. Somewhat baffled, I said "ok, sounds good".

As part of the class warm up period, we were introduced to something called "tai chi"; specifically Lee Ying Arng's modified Tai Chi form. I had never seen nor heard of such a thing; and as a traditionally athletic teenager, the slow and gentle movements were frustratingly awkward, and immensely difficult. Thankfully, I was surrounded by several other university students and teachers, young and old who were also stumbling through the postures with me!

Upon returning to school in the Fall of 1979, I was given a book by a fellow tai chi student and University Professor of Anthropology. He had run across it in a book store while studying the native American culture in Oklahoma during his summer break. The book was entitled "T'ai Chi Ch'uan for Health and Self-Defense" by T.T. Liang.

After graduating from university in the summer of 1982 my wife Kim and I got married, started our professional careers, had a couple children, and got on with living the American Dream. During it all, the notion of this "tai chi" would continue to pop up like a shimmering mirage. Resolved to do more, I haphazardly began to search for knowledgable instructors. Signing up for community education classes, chatting up random gym class coaches, and quizzing miscellaneous fitness instructors proved to be underwhelming and unsatisfactory. Discouraged, I would pull out my copy of "T'ai Chi Ch'uan for Health and Self-Defense" to see if by magic, some simple instructional illustrations might yet appear on the pages.

In the summer of 1992 we moved to Rochester, Minnesota.

Sometime during the Fall of 1995 I was pushing a cart full of groceries through the check out lane and happened to notice a copy of Mpls.St.Paul Magazine staring at me from the end cap. On the front cover was the image of an older Chinese gentleman with a caption about acupuncture. An idea forming, I grabbed the magazine and added it to the cart.

Back at home, I enthusiastically read through the magazine article with the certainty that this doctor of Chinese Medicine, living in the Twin Cities, will know of a credible tai chi instructor. Even more serendipitously, the doctor's contact information was listed in the article (keep in mind, this was WAY before the internet).

After respectfully introducing myself on the phone, I explained why I was calling, and what I was looking for. The doctor briefly went silent while he considered my query, and then he announced, "I know of a young tai chi master in Saint Paul who you should contact. I don't know his number, but his name is Ray Hayward."

Now with a solid lead to pursue, it was time to invoke: 555-1212; in other words, calling the ubiquitous number for directory assistance to ask for the number(s) for a "Ray Hayward".

After receiving the number from the operator and making the call, I was finally able to connect with the target of my search.

"Is this Mr. Ray Hayward?"

"Yes."

"My name is Mike Cain, and I am interested in tai chi, do you teach tai chi?"

"Yes."

"How can I get started in one of your classes?"

"You live in Rochester right? I teach in Northfield on Saturday mornings. Call Renee for more information."

"Thank you sir."

<click>

On a Saturday morning in November 1995, I made the one hour drive up to Northfield, MN and walked into the Arts Guild building to formally introduce myself and join the class.

For the next several Saturdays, it was unlearn, relearn, and try to relax. Adding to the struggle, I had to pay attention to enough detail so I could practice the movements after my one hour drive back to Rochester. On one particular Saturday morning, I got up enough courage to ask Ray if he had ever heard of a book called, "T'ai Chi Ch'uan for Health and Self-Defense" by T.T. Liang. After a thoughtful pause, a devious smile appeared, and a profound answer was given: "Sure, he's my teacher."

For the next few years I attended class in Northfield on Saturdays and sometimes Sundays. During these morning workouts, our class enthusiastically bantered while working through the tai chi long form, and then the sword form - something by the way that was only rumored to even exist.

On more than one occasion, there would be me, one other student, and Ray. At the time, the fact that our esteemed teacher would invest a valuable Saturday morning to instruct only a couple newbies was a total shock to me. Later I came to realize that sincerity and devotion to his students were sustaining hallmarks of Master Ray Hayward.

At some point the number of students attending the weekly Northfield classes dropped to an unsustainable level. I was simultaneously humbled and honored when Master Hayward pulled me aside after class and told me the news that he would no longer be able to teach in Northfield. He then lightly suggested I could visit the Saint Paul studio to continue my lessons privately if I was so interested.

Over the course of several years, I traveled up to the Studio every few months to meet, talk, and receive profound lessons in the science and art of tai chi. On many occasions, Master Hayward would pull out the ever present "T'ai Chi Ch'uan for Health and Self-Defense" by T.T. Liang" and announce with big smile, "Look here, there's the answer written out for you." Still no illustrations by the way.

During one of my seasonal visits to the Studio, it was suggested that a tai chi class in Rochester should be formed. Boy was I excited; the one and only Ray Hayward gonna teach in Rochester!

I was surprised to learn that he really wanted ME to teach, and my protests to the contrary were parried with the statement, "to teach is to learn twice". After more discussion and planning, I said I needed a teaching partner. The immediate response was, "Done, I have a guy!"

During the summer months of 2007 I met with Dominick Veldman, and along with my wife Kim we started to put together a plan for the start of the Med City Tai Chi Club. The commitment, investment, and dedication put forth by our dear friend Dominick are a testament to the vision and leadership of Master Hayward. To teach alongside a knowledgable partner is to learn thrice!

For more than two decades I traveled around the world as an IBM database consultant. During this time I met with hundreds of different companies and many diverse clients. I also took on a personal mission to test, refine, and ultimately make use of the principles embodied in the tai chi. From the experience, I can report that what has been so graciously shared by Master Hayward is both efficient and effective when leading business engagements. A secret weapon if you will. The techniques manifested mentally during individual and group interaction are just as potent and advantageous as they are when used physically on the hardwood floor. This revelation, more than anything else was an unexpected surprise, and a source of motivation.

As an example, the following scenario reveals what I ultimately labeled as "care and not care". When physically practicing pushing hands, it is important to care enough to provide a good push, but not care if that push affects your partner. When consulting, it is important to care enough to provide good advice, but not care if the client refuses to take it. This is at the heart of what it means to be a good partner; and good partners are golden!

On the many drives to and from Northfield, to and from Saint Paul, to and from our own classes, I continue to reflect and ruminate on the arc of my tai chi experiences. The analogy I keep coming back to goes like this...

There is a magnificent mansion surrounded by immaculate gardens and towering trees. Walking past, one is immediately in awe of the sight. A feeling of mystery and intrigue emanates from the property. Curiosity abounds. Suddenly, the front door opens, and a gentleman smiles, waves, and invites you to walk up and join him on the extraordinary front porch. A cup of coffee is served. After sitting a spell, he opens the massive front door, and asks if you'd like to see inside. Walking into the dimly lit foyer, he says, wait, let me switch on a light so you can see properly. What appears before your eyes is virtually indescribable; beauty and craftsmanship at the highest level. After a while, he invites you down the hall to the next room, switching on other lights. Once again, more examples of bewildering beauty and craftsmanship. And so it goes, for as long as you can keep up. Room after exquisite room is illuminated, shared, explained.

To sum up, allow me to share this from one of my many discussions with the late, great Master G. (aka Mr. Paul Gallagher)… if you had to name the top five most influential people during your life, not counting your parents, who would they be, and why? Ray Hayward is on my list. And now you know why.

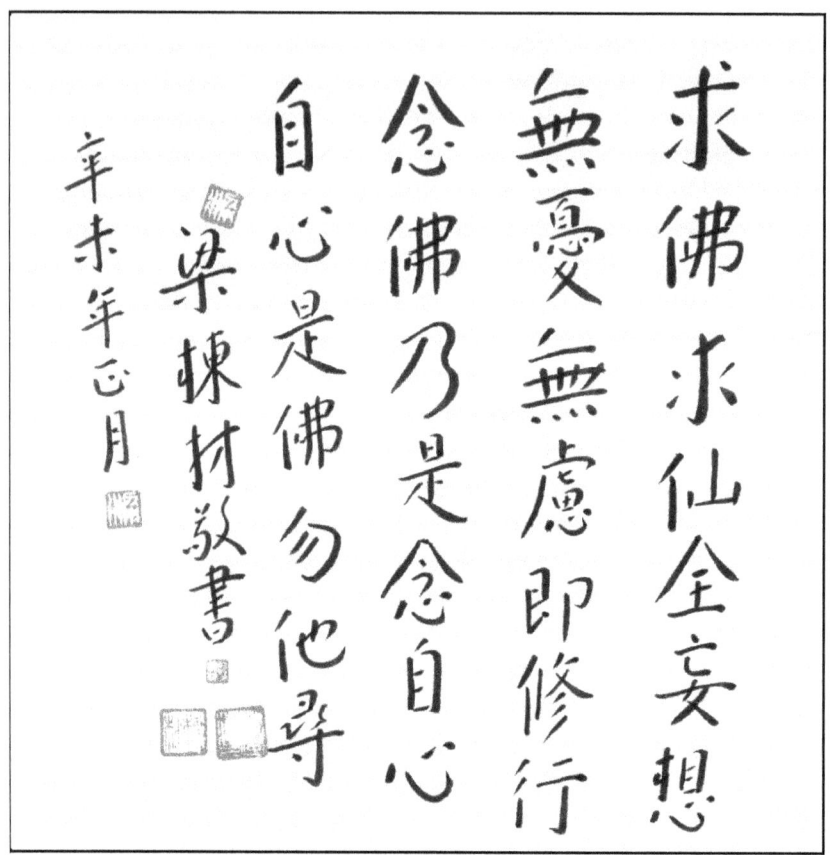

To seek Buddhahood or to seek Immortality - both are illusions.

To have neither grief nor care - that is practicing Cultivation.

To contemplate Buddha is to contemplate your own heart-mind.

Your own heart-mind is Buddha; do not seek anything else.

Respectfully written by Liang Tung Ts'ai

Translation by Master Paul B. Gallagher

Karen Deley

I met Ray Hayward in January of 1987, at a Hsingi workshop in Winnipeg, Manitoba, Canada. I then started to commute to Minnesota, to continue my learning from Ray, which included Yang style Taiji solo form, Chi Kung, weapons, and the animal form. I then became an instructor and taught under Ray Haywards supervision in Winnipeg, Manitoba, Canada, and organized workshops on his behalf. Taiji changed my life, and continues to be a part of it as of today.

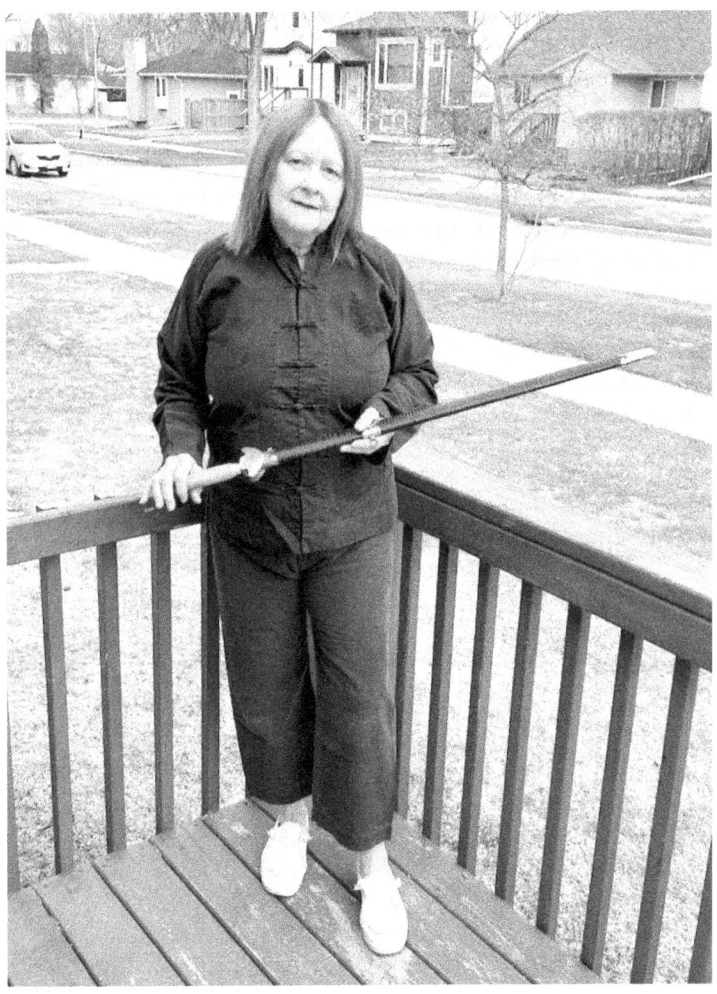

Julie Cisler

A Great Teacher

"The best teacher in the world is someone who loves what he or she does, and just loves it in front of you." ~ Fred Rogers

I am humbled to be asked to contribute to this book. It is perhaps because I have had the great fortune to study with Sifu Ray Hayward for decades. I am filled with gratitude at the opportunity I've had to be in his classes. He has taught me more than I can remember about Taijiquan. But he has also taught me many important life lessons.

Sifu Hayward has been dedicated to refining and mastering the art of Taijiquan. He studied diligently with all of his teachers, especially Master T.T. Liang and Grandmaster Wai-lun Choi. He transmits their important lessons to all of his students. Sifu Hayward has been a font of knowledge, and for this I have great confidence that the arts I have learned from my teacher adhere to the principles of the Classics.

But Sifu Ray Hayward is so much more than a dedicated practitioner; I have also seen him striving with the same energy and attention to detail to develop and refine his teaching methods. He has been careful to transmit the methods that he has learned from his teachers. In addition, he shares with all of us the refinements to the methods he learned, as well as new teaching methods he has developed, in order to reach as many students as possible.

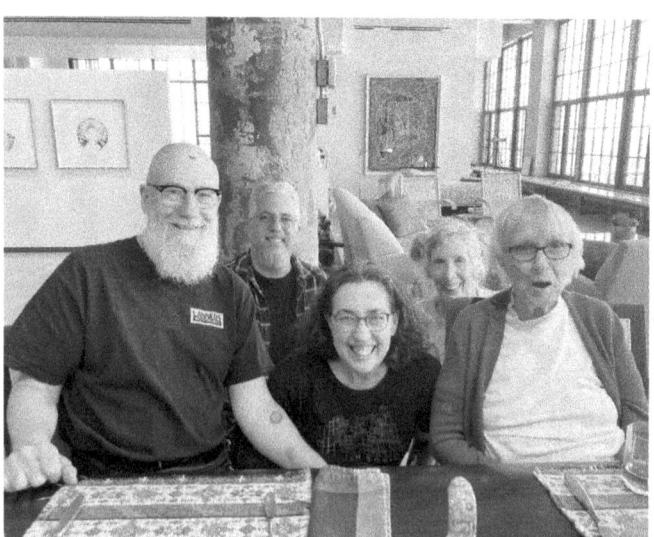

Sifu Hayward has taught this awkward and slow student more

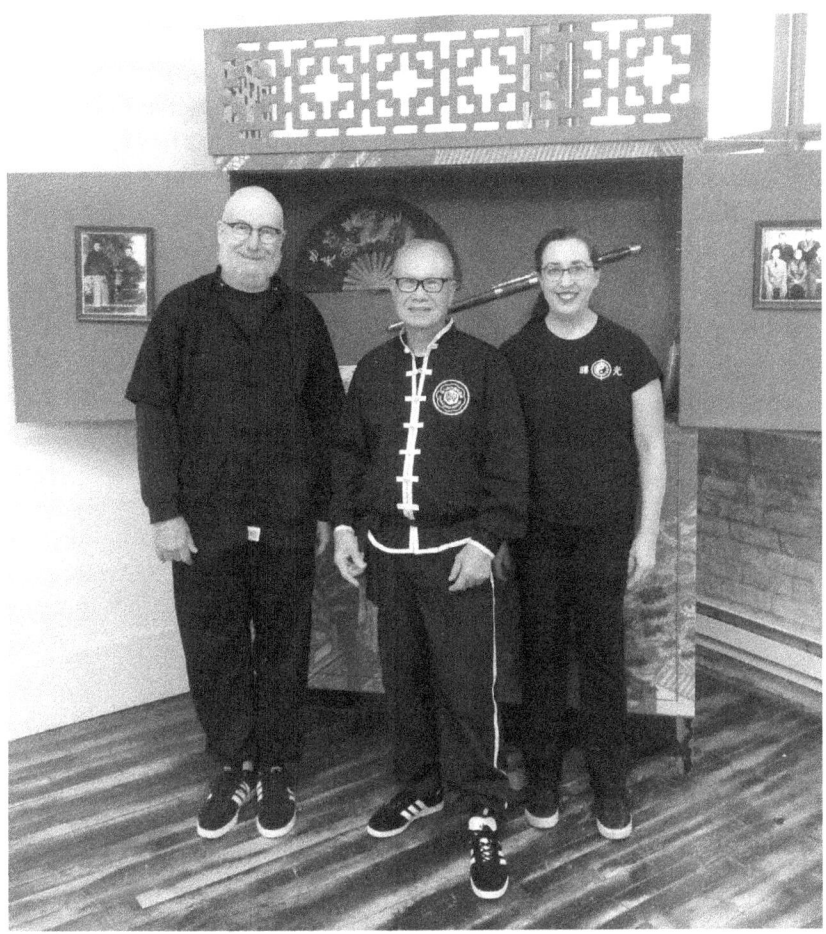

forms and practices than I can remember. He has also instilled in me more confidence and compassion for myself and others.

One of my proudest moments happened when we visited Master Choi at his school in Chicago. Sifu Choi asked our group to practice the Baguazhang Mother Palms form of Chang Chao-tung. When we finished, Sifu Choi said to me, "I have a correction for your teacher, because I know you are his student." What a great compliment from the Grandmaster! It warms my heart to this day.

Thank you, Sifu!

Diane Cannon

My name is Diane Cannon and I have been a student of T'ai Chi Ch'uan since 1987. You see, my life was a bit hectic back then, and I was looking for a practice to calm and center my spirit. Three very clear signs led me to a T'ai Chi class at the Chrysalis Center in Wilmington, Delaware, where I was living at the time. I had an immediate connection to the practice of Chi Kung and the Solo Form and before I knew it, a year had passed. My teacher spoke often of his teacher, Sifu Ray Hayward, and brought him in to offer us a weekend workshop. I was already experiencing the meditative and centering benefits of Chi Kung and the Solo Form, but when Sifu Ray Hayward shared his experience in the art, his depth of knowledge, his joyful spirit and love of the complete system of the Yang Style T'ai Chi forms and training - I was hooked! I continued studying with my current teacher for another two years during which I had the pleasure of many more workshops with Sifu Ray. Then in 1990, I approached Sifu Ray and asked if he would accept me as his student. His response was an immediate "yes" and our T'ai Chi journey began!

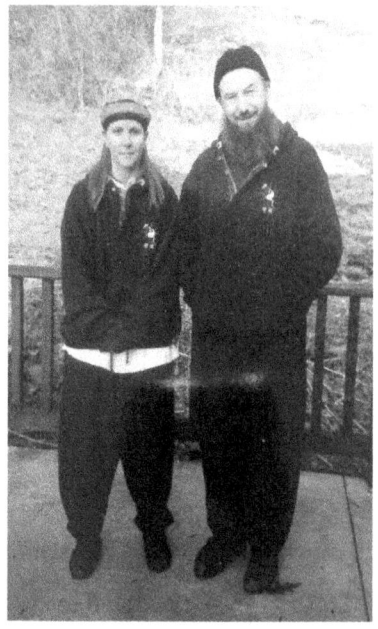

One of the first things Sifu Ray wanted me to do was offer a T'ai Chi class to women. I was shocked and unprepared and did not feel worthy to begin teaching. He pushed me hard to do so. When it comes to T'ai Chi, Sifu has a way of knowing what you need and what you are ready for before you do, so between my trust in his wisdom and desire to follow his request, I began a women's class out of my home. And let me tell you, how I grew: as practitioner/student, and teacher!

I soon found myself in love with the Art of T'ai Chi Ch'uan so much, that I wanted to know it all - meditation, solo forms, weapons, two person forms, pushing hands, - I couldn't get enough. I traveled to Minneapolis to train with him in the small basement school on University Ave., then to Ann Arbor, MI while he was there. There we trained the Chen-style Taiji Canon Fist Form and more! We worked out in a beautiful park and his joy of teaching was infectious! See, that's the thing with studying with Sifu, he makes learning fun. When he sees you are interested and serious, he will work you

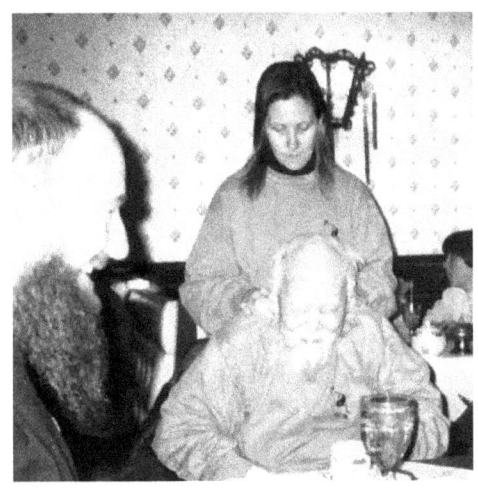

hard, push you just the right amount, and then the mental pushing hands begins! I do believe he got that from our Master, T.T. Liang, with whom I had the honor of knowing and loving!

In around 1993, Sifu Ray moved back to the Twin Cities in MN and I made a commitment to travel to train with him for a ten day period twice a year. In addition to my travel to his school, I brought him out east for workshops and yearly retreats (some years we would have two retreats/year). At the end of each retreat, we would take the students to visit Master Liang. Sifu always wanted to share the complete art, the familia aspect of being a student of T'ai Chi, which to this day I honor and pass on to my students. He taught me, in a very subtle way, the familia traditions, the unspoken ways of being with your Master, your teacher, your students, what I like to call "the quiet actions of a serious T'ai Chi Practitioner". See, in addition to his excitement when he teaches, he is also watching you, seeing

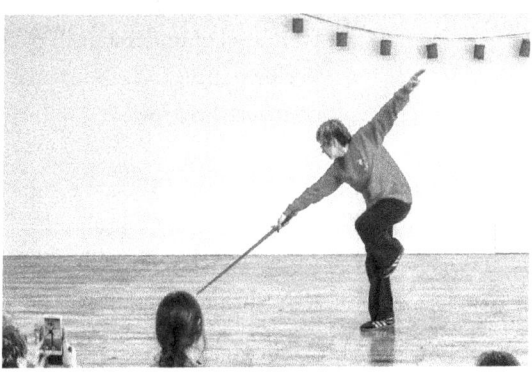

what you are paying attention to when it comes to respect on the floor when training, when dining out with students and teachers, how you interact with your students, etc. I only hope I have honored Master Liang

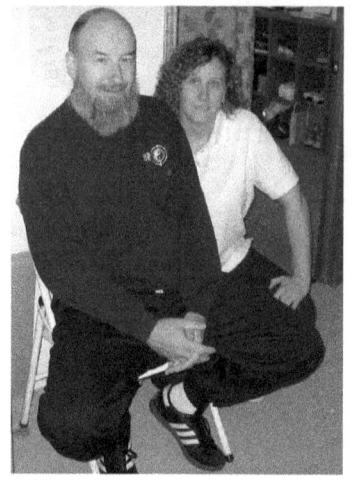

and Sifu Ray in continuing this practice and teaching,

During this time of traveling to MN and private lessons when I brought him out East, Sifu shared his expertise in other styles as well. As he taught me the complete Yang Family System of T'ai Chi, he wanted to expose me to other methods and styles. If you want to learn and train, he will teach! He taught me forms and training practices in Baguazhang, Xingyiquan, Praying Mantis, and Li Ho Pa Fa! His ability to not only understand various styles, but also to translate the information in a way that you understand and manifest is impeccable! Many teachers can do, not all can teach…Sifu has mastered both! So much is learned from being pushed outside your comfort zone to demonstrate/teach/give a talk, whatever method is needed, he is sensitive to your needs as a student and will walk thru the challenge with you. He requested

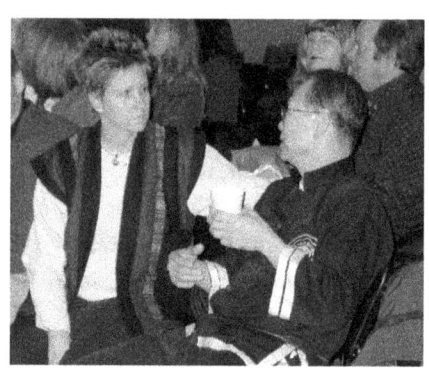

demonstrations from me at many of his Chinese New Year Demonstrations, demonstrations from not only me, but my students at all the retreats I hosted. When this happens, you pick up your sword and perform, and your level of understanding, performance, and confidence continues to grow!

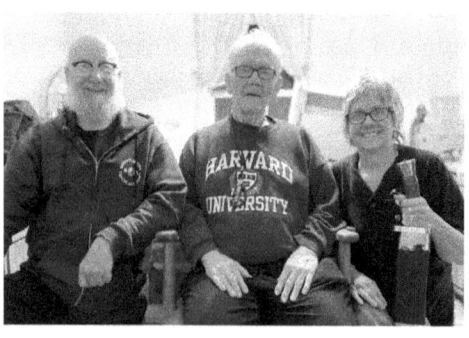

In the mid 1990's, I established my T'ai Chi school, Ming Tao T'ai Chi Ch'uan. In addition to regular daytime and evening classes,

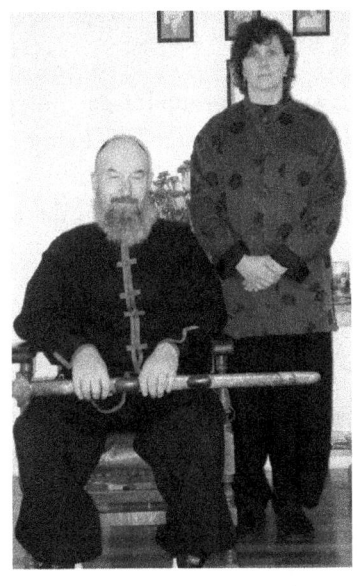

private lessons, and seminars, I have had the honor of hosting Sifu many times as well as Master Wai Lun Choi!

Sifu's generosity in sharing all aspects of all the martial arts he has studied over the years is beyond my expectations of any teacher. He truly takes the position that "there are no secrets". He gives freely of his knowledge and understanding of each art and is more than happy to share his many teachers if you prove worthy! He shared Master Liang with me, Master Choi, and Master Paul Gallagher, a true blessing. Sifu honors his relationships with his fellow classmates and dedicated students, and will go over and beyond what any student would expect. My suggestion, just honor "the quiet actions of a serious T'ai Chi Practitioner".

In 1998, Sifu accepted me as a 7th generation disciple. It was an honor to be initiated into our lineage and I have been truly blessed. How can I summarize what it has been like to study with such a knowledgeable, dedicated, generous Master of the Arts? I know this, he has taught me to have fun in the learning, to grow in confidence in training, to think critically about what is going on in each movement, to be respectful of the art, the teachers, and the students, to push outside my comfort zone, to embrace growth, love of the arts, and most of all - have fun. Being a part of our lineage is a true honor, and it has been a blessing to initiate two of my most dedicated students as 8th generation disciples in October 2021. Only with Sifu's support, encouragement, and dedication to me as a student, could these achievements be possible. With all respect, dedication and love, to you Sir, I give a bow from the waist.

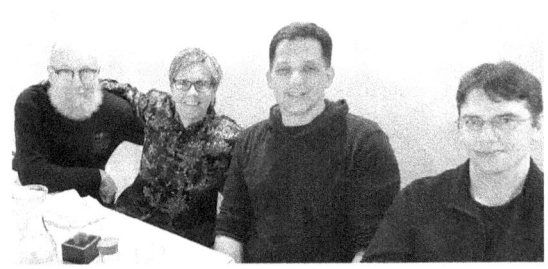

Frederick Sparks

In August of 1987, I was invited to attend a private group lesson conducted by Ray Hayward, a student at the time of Master T.T. Liang, in St Paul, MN. Little did we know that this chance encounter would lead to our 37-year relationship as teacher and student and a most valued friendship.

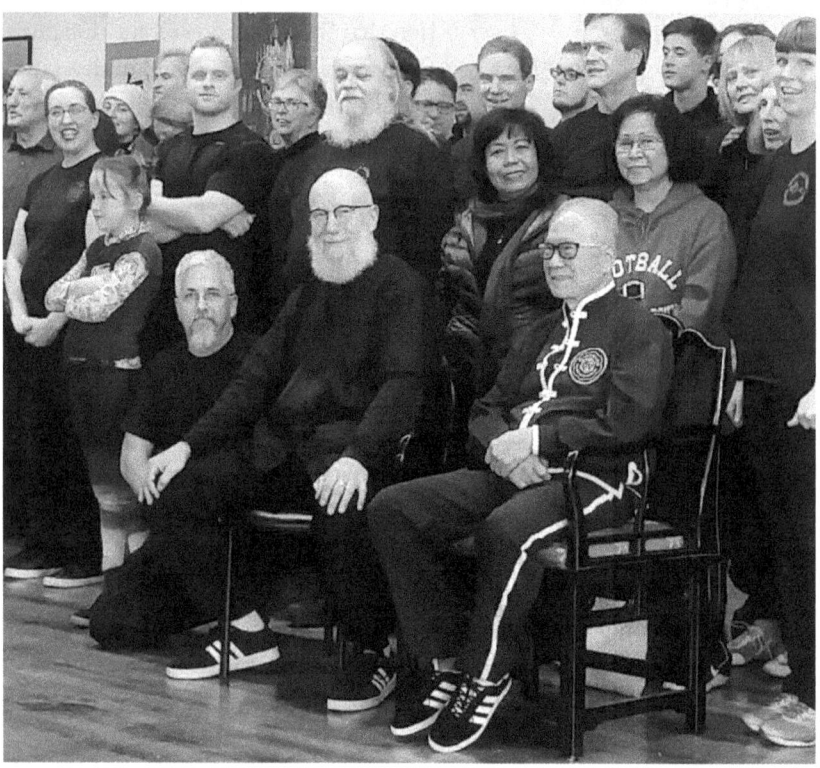

Back then, Sifu Ray adhered to the "old fashioned" style of teaching of his teachers—specifically that the student had to earn the teacher's trust over time by the student demonstrating good character in their personal life and a practice ethic in their study before deeper knowledge, training methods, and applications were shared with the student. This was and is a point of integrity within all the lineages Sifu Ray has studied. Consequently, I studied for 4 years, learning the Yang Family Long solo form and Tai Chi Cane, Sword, Saber and Staff, before I was given permission to attend my first pushing hands classes at his school.

I will never forget the feeling of being both captivated and intimidated by the skills of his senior students at the time, and, in my own innocent lack of knowledge, discovering a world of inherited skill sets within Sifu Ray that I had only read about but didn't know could—or even did—exist in anyone. He had cataloged, practiced, and inherited everything Master Liang offered him, which was a lifetime of study and practice among the best teachers of the 20th century, complimented by additional studies under his teacher Dr Leung Kay-chi and Sifu Lo Man-biu.

In those days, Sifu Ray instructed us to learn about hard styles that he had studied to complement the Tai Chi practices, just as T.T. Liang instructed him to do. The next several years were a humbling experience, full of learning, commitment, personal development, fellowship, and the joy of a fully rounded practice with Sifu Ray and his many students.

It was during this period that Sifu Ray met and developed his relationship with the great Grandmaster Wai Lun Choi, who, in short, brought everything full circle and in focus for Sifu Rays' lifetime of study, and fully cultivated him as the highly skilled practitioner and teacher that he is today. I am profoundly grateful for the generosity of Master T.T. Liang, Grandmaster Choi, Master Gin foon Mark, and all of his teachers for everything they taught and shared with Sifu Ray, which he now makes readily available for any person who is willing to put in the time and effort to learn and practice.

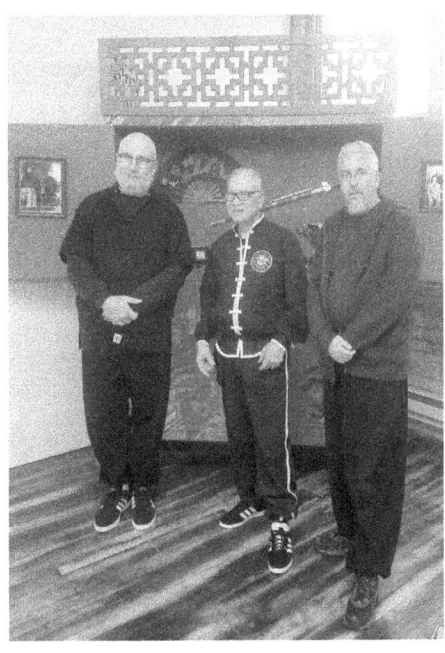

Thank you.
Frederick Sparks
April 25th, 2024

Robert "Bob" Klanderud

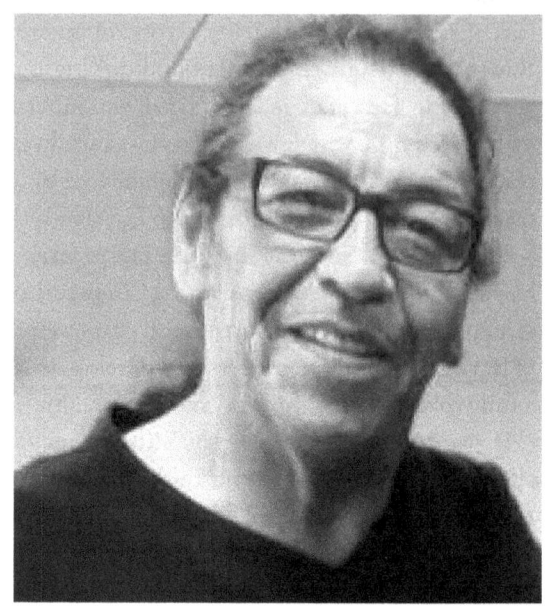

Hau Misun and hello my younger wiser brother!!! So good to hear about your 40th book. I am living in remote California and have to go some distance to get interweb and I apologize for the late response. Ray, I would have to mention the great inspiration I have received from you and the way that you have integrated Tai Chi into your everyday life, Tai Chi as a way of life!!!

I really enjoy the Inspired Teacher when I think of you very often. I still owe you the Sacred Name and look forward to presenting it to you brother. My Name is Ahkisha Oka Wicasa, the man who makes a sound for the people!!! Love you Brother!

James Postiglione

Celebrating Sifu Ray Hayward 40 Years of Teaching
By James Postiglione, long-time student, 7th generation disciple

My Tai Chi experience with Sifu Ray started in the late 1980's. I had previously learned the Yang style short form from Sean Marshal and was a few months into learning the Kuang Ping form from Marillyn Alyssum when a classmate mentioned Sifu Ray's school. I was intrigued by the number of classes per week and the different styles taught so I went to check it out the next Tuesday. This class was a small group of advanced students, but Sifu Ray let me give it a try. I was impressed by the students skill and softness and I was hooked. I have had the good fortune of learning from Sifu Ray since then and have benefited from the generous way he passes on guidance he received from many teachers and many hours of practice. It has been a great journey to observe and experience Sifu Ray's ever growing martial and teaching skill.

Tai Chi is a big part of my life and has improved my health greatly. Most days begin with warmups, meditation and a round of the long form, its like a mini vacation. I enjoy the calm, flowing movement, it is so peaceful but also enhances the senses like feeling connection to the ground, the way wind cuts past my limbs and how the solitude reveals the slightest sounds.

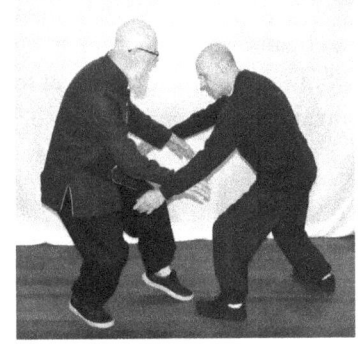

Study with Sifu Ray has given me the opportunity to teach others as a helper or substitute instructor and later in leading my own class. I am so thankful for the opportunity to teach, it's a great way to help others as well as deepening ones level of understanding. It is a great pleasure to observe students become more relaxed, fluid and healthy. Teaching also provides so many ways to improve; like analyzing your form as you demonstrate, explaining the classics and researching questions that you cannot answer right away. I feel very privileged to pass on Sifu Ray's teaching and am so thankful for the opportunity.

Thank you Sifu Ray!

Bryan Davis

I met Ray at a seminar he was giving in Delaware shortly after he had moved to Minnesota. He was 24 and I was 18, and we hit it off right away. After all, we were young, and everyone else at the seminar was so old; they must have been something like 35 years old or even older. Ray immediately started calling me "Young Man", and so I started calling him "Old Man". The two-day seminar focused on Pushing Hands, and for the first day (that is, for two 4-hour sessions), we did nothing but Willow Bends. Ray made sure to do Willow with everyone that was there. This was in the fall of 1984. My teacher at the time really wanted to learn the Two-Person Dance of Master Liang, and since he needed a partner, I volunteered. We learned a little bit during that seminar and made arrangements to visit Ray in Minnesota the following winter. I had been doing T'ai Chi for about 2 years by the time we visited in February, but after that 10-day visit, I was hooked for life.

Going forward, I would visit Ray a couple times a year for a week or so, sleeping on the floor of his boarding house. We talked about T'ai Chi all night and worked out for 10 hours a day — every day — for the duration of my stay. I learned a pile of forms from T'ai Chi, Pa Kua, Hsing-I, Shaolin and more. I got to meet so many great people through this relationship

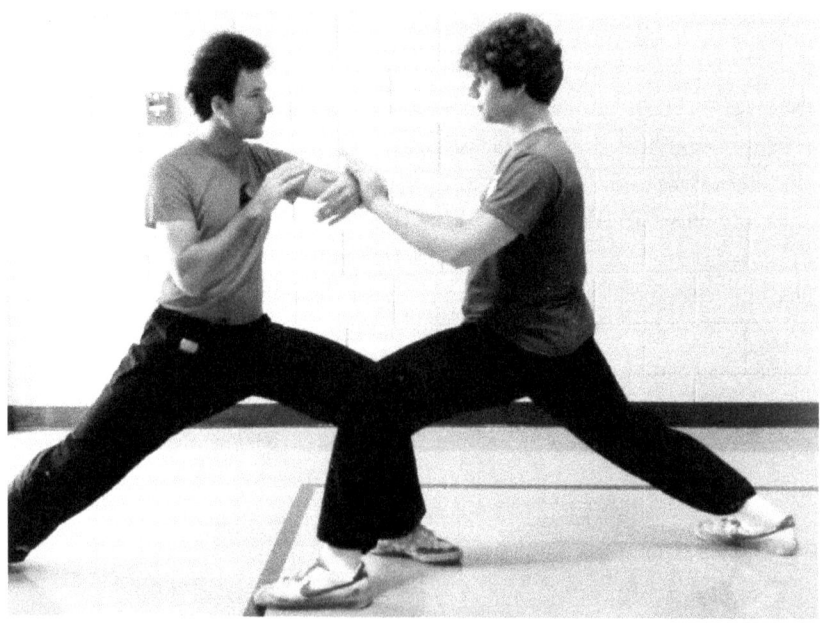

as well: Master Liang, Paul Gallagher, Ken Cohen, Leung Kay Chi, Mrs. Hayward (Ray's mom), and more. By this time, I was teaching my own classes back in Delaware. I would sponsor Ray to come East for a couple seminars each year, which were always good. My students always enjoyed his visits. Ray still comes out to my school to give seminars and this year we are starting the retreats back up again. It should be great.

So, I have been studying with Ray for the 40 years he has lived in Minnesota. From the beginning we developed a friendship, but since then, Ray and I have become more than friends; we are brothers. He is part of my family, and I am part of his. I have learned an incredible amount from him over the years and had the pleasure of passing that along to my students. I am a disciple. Being part of this great lineage is an honor. My relationship with Ray and with T'ai Chi has absolutely changed my life.

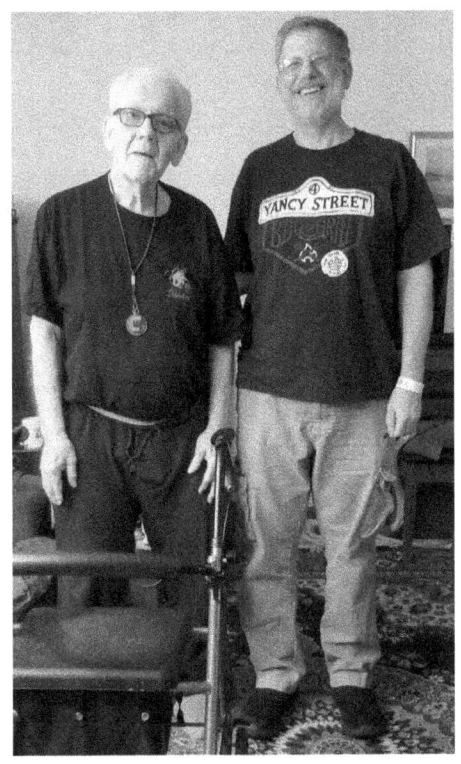

Bryan Davis (right), with Paul Gallagher (left).

Thank you,
Bryan

Sifu Speaks

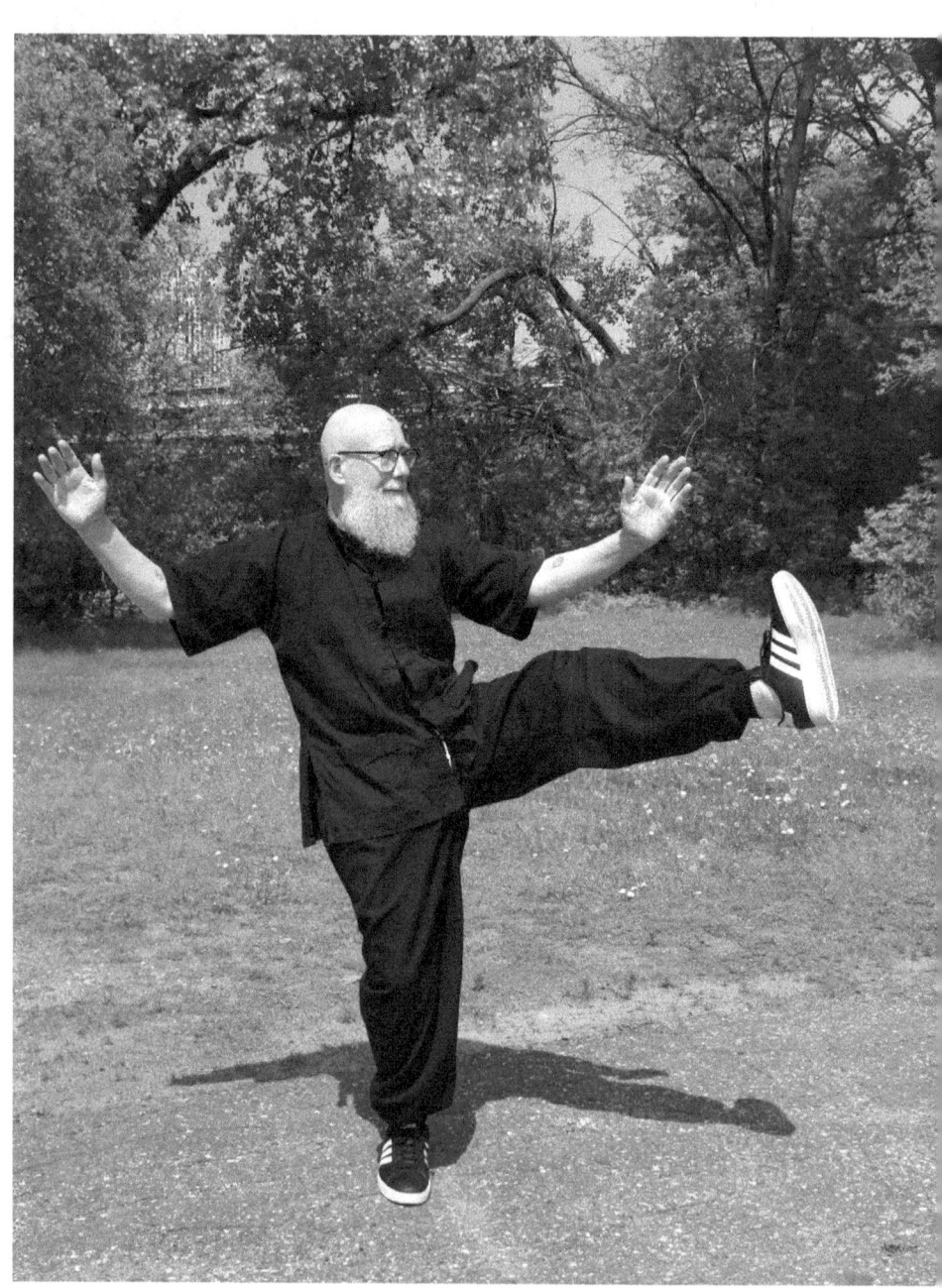

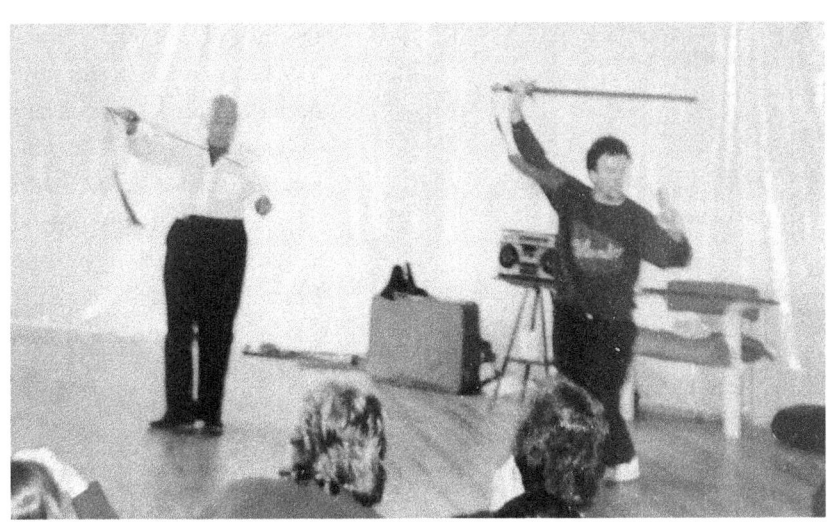

Introduction to 40th Anniversary Book
by Ray Hayward

"Teachers teach students, students teach students, students teach teachers."
~ Chinese Proverb

July 29th marks forty years that I have been living and teaching in Minnesota. I was born in Massachusetts and met and studied with Master T.T. Liang in Boston from 1977 to 1981. Master Liang "retired" in 1981 and move to Minnesota to be with his daughter, An Le. I stayed in Massachusetts and studied with the late Sifu Lo Man-biu in 1982, and with the late Dr Leung Kay-chi from 1979 to 1984, both in Boston.

In addition to learning Taiji from Master Liang, he also taught me how to teach. After I had learned the Form and had a good foundation, Master Liang would assign a new student to me in each class and have me teach them some postures or techniques. At the end of the class, Liang would come over and offer corrections to the student, and then critique my

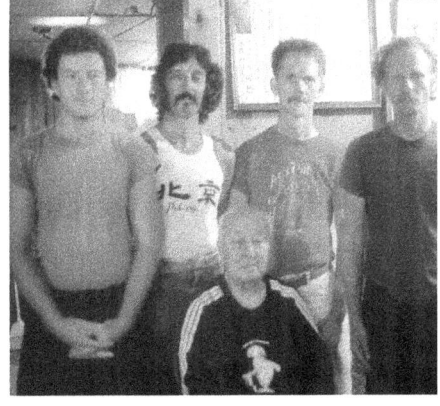

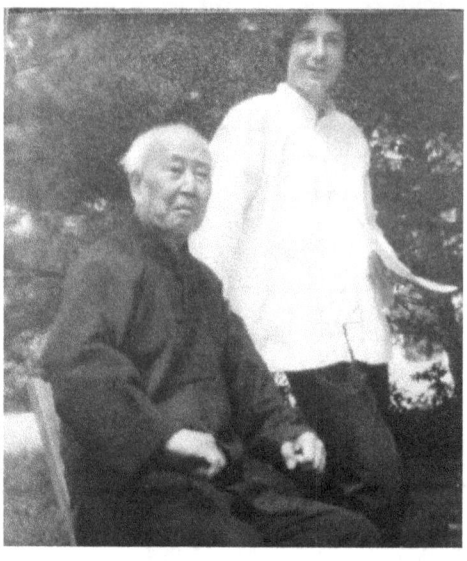

teaching or give me hints and tips about [teach]ing the material. In this way I was an ass[istant] under Master Liang and helped in his cl[asses].

I assisted Master Liang for a weeklong seminar at the Omega Institute in 1979. Master Liang also gave me my first teach[ing] assignment, teaching by myself, at the N[ew] England School of Acupuncture. I learne[d] a lot about teaching and learning from th[ose] experiences and Liang's guidance. His ap[]proach to teaching opened yet another fa[cet of] my Taiji journey. All this put me on the p[ath] of teaching and learning, and this turned [out] to be my vocation, even teaching seminar[s and] workshops on teaching and learning Taij[i].

"In learning you will teach, and in teaching, you will learn."
~ Phil Collins

After he moved from Boston, I kept in contact with Master Liang through letters an[d] occasional phone calls. Then in late 1983 I heard rumors that Liang had come out of r[etire]ment and was teaching again. I decided to visit him for a week in January of 1984. I lea[rned] more on that visit than in the previous three years. I immediately made plans to go bac[k and] visit in May of 1984. I spent three weeks in May living and studying with Master Lian[g at] his home in St Cloud, MN.

"When you learn, teach. When you get, give."
~ Maya Angelou

During that three-week visit, I met many of Master Liang's, students and assisted hi[m in] his classes. He told his students that they learned most of his forms but didn't get his P[ush]ing Hands and applications. He said they could learn those aspects from me. Many to[ok] ang up on the offer and I got to introduce Pushing Hands to many of my classmates. M[aster] Liang suggested that I move to Minnesota to finish my studies with him and teach Pus[hing] Hands, and applications. He also said to teach the other styles and weapons I was prac[ticing] at that time such as Xingyi, Bagua, Northern Praying Mantis, Shaolin, and Qinna, as [well] as spear, staff, double daggers, three section staff, and fighting and fencing sets.

I went back home, gave notice at work, settled all my affairs, and prepared to go to M[innesota].

sota. One of the best decisions of my life! I came with a sword, saber, spear, cane, some books and clothes, 393.00 dollars in my pocket, and bucketfuls of hopes and dreams. I taught at the East River Flats Park most of the Summer and into the Fall. Many of my students were Master Liang's students who lived in the Twin Cities. I taught four nights a week and Saturday 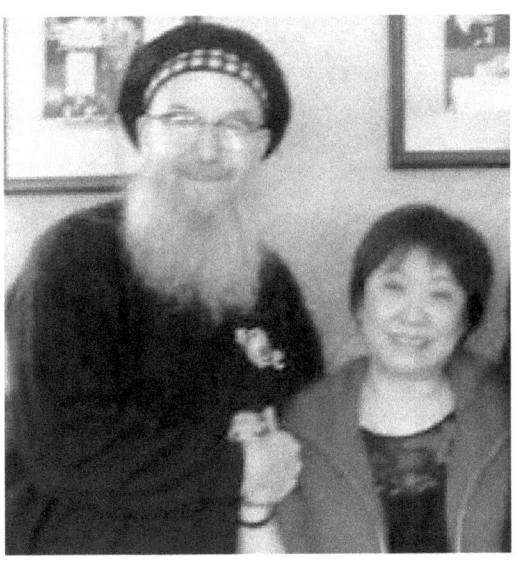 mornings without missing any classes due to the weather.

When the weather turned cold, but mostly because it was getting dark early, I looked for an inside space to teach and practice. My classmate and practice partner, Jonah Friedman, had a beautiful studio in St Paul, the Twin Cities Tai Chi Chuan Studio, near Highway 280. He traded me two nights a week to teach my classes in return for me teaching and practicing with him privately. Later, Jonah's life took some major changes, and I took over the whole studio.

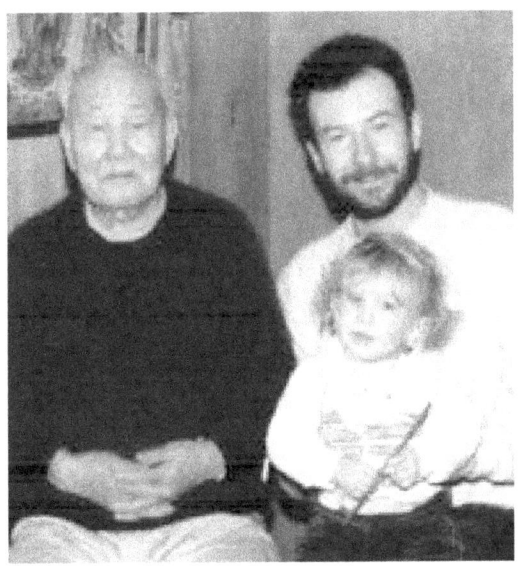

I moved to the Hampden building in 1988 and had a basement studio for a few years. Joanne Von Blon, my disciple, offered to make the studio a nonprofit and give me a regular salary and benefits. Classes moved from the basement to the 2nd floor in 1993, we

73

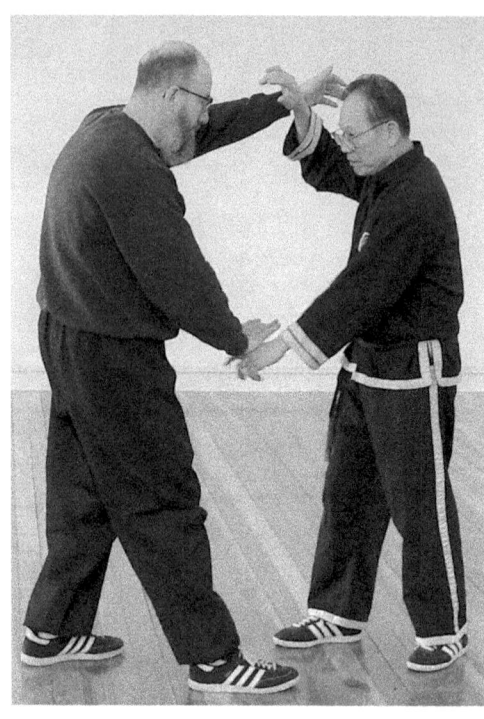

installed a gorgeous wood floor, and there, six days a week, I taught my guts out! In 2016 I opened my own studio, Mindful Motion Taiji Academy, and taught at the Ivy Building until Covid and the Minneapolis Riots closed that space down in the spring of 2020. Burned the roof actually!

"My practice is for my students; my teaching is for me."
~ Unknown

After the lockdown was lifted, during which I learned about Zoom, YouTube, and Patreon, I returned to teaching in the park, renting space at our current home at St Sahag to teach in person, and teaching online. I've tried to retire, or semi-retire, but Taiji and teaching are in my blood. I get so much from sharing my discoveries from my personal practice. I also learn tons from my students' practice, research, and their "ahas!" On my 60th birthday I handed over the running of the school to my long-time student and disciple, Julie Cisler, one of the editors and the designer of this, and all my books.

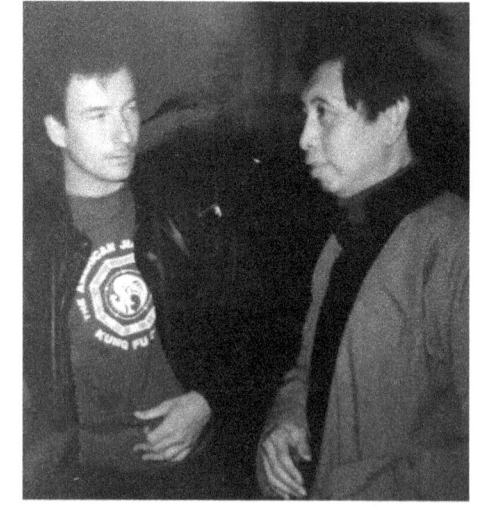

"The highest level isn't showing others what you can do. The highest level is teaching others to do what you can do."
~ Naqshbandi Sufi teaching

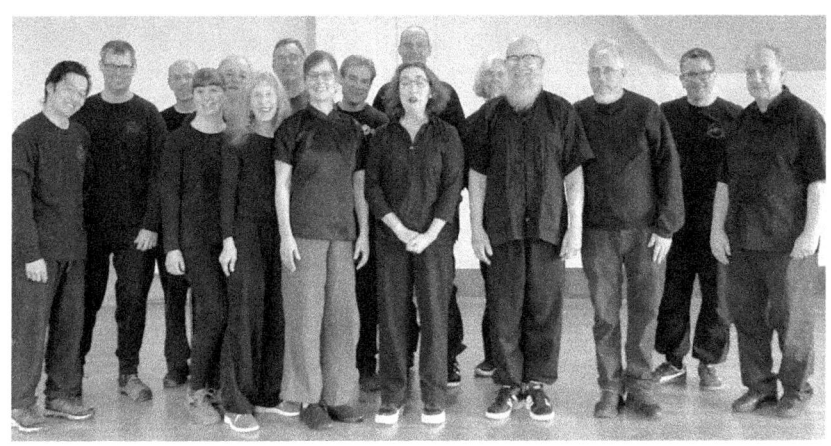

Through the decades, I not only used my own learning, practice, and teaching as my laboratory, I studied many methods and schools of thought on teaching and learning. Sufism gave me many great ideas about how we can learn. Hypnotherapy taught me many useful ideas on how to arrange my words so the message I wanted to convey would get through and not be derailed. Teaching, together with learning and practicing, became my craft.

I used my experience to learn how to play the drums at age 38, and even learned to read drum music. I saw the parallel in so many aspects of our lives where the correct methods would help with any kind of learning, teaching, or practice. I can safely say that there are universal principles, concepts, and theories to teaching and learning that lead to achievement. If they are not followed, the results will fall short. Of course, as my other teacher, Grandmaster Wai-lun Choi says, "There are no guarantees."

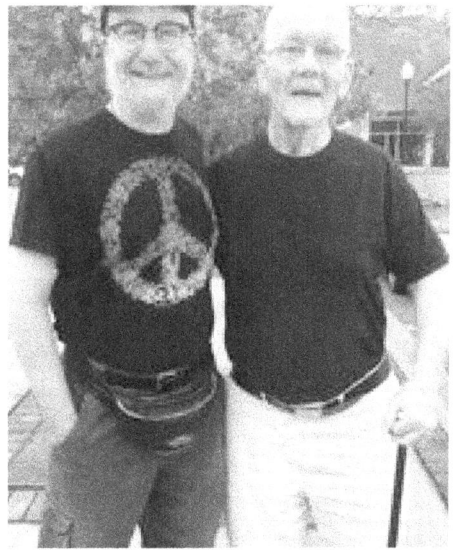

"My heart is singing for joy this morning! A miracle has happened! The light of understanding has shone upon my little pupil's mind (Helen Keller), and behold, all things are changed!"
~ Anne Sullivan Macy

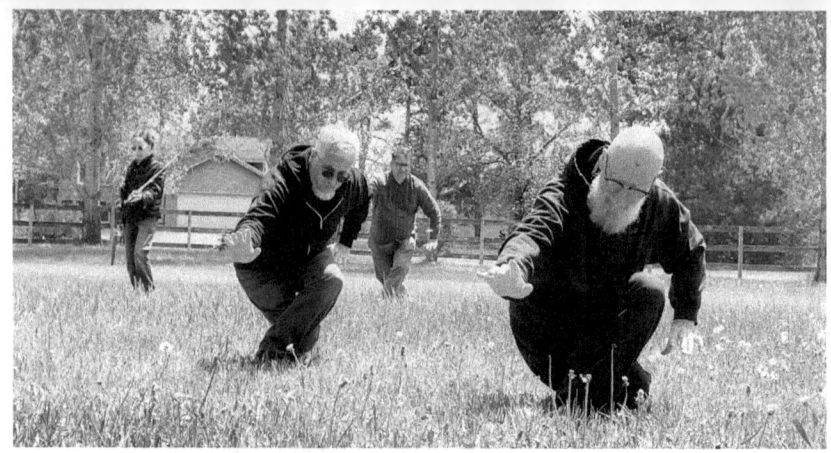

In addition to seminars and workshops on the East Coast, I taught at many places around the Twin Cities. I spread Master T.T. Liang's message, "Taiji is the Whole World's Exercise." Here are a few:

Sister Kenney Pain Clinic at Abbott Northwestern Hospital
General Mills World Headquarters
Courage Center
University of Minnesota, MPLS campus
Virginia Piper Cancer Center
Zenon Dance Company
The Marsh
Minnesota ALS Association
Hazelden
Evolve Fitness
Northwestern Health Sciences
MNDOT
Center Point/ MN Shiatsu Center
Pillsbury R and D Headquarters
Macalester College
Semaphore Dance Company
Minnesota Homeschooler's Alliance
MN Veterans Home
Bush Foundation
Carleton College

I'd like to share with you two of my teaching/learning experiences:

When I first began teaching in Minnesota, the students would ask questions. There were many I could answer, but there was an equal amount I couldn't. I would take these questions to my private class in St Cloud and get Master Liang's answer. I began writing the questions down, putting my idea or answer below, then writing Liang's answer below mine, to bring back to tell the student. I could see where my answers were either far off, or partially correct, or correct. I began to see where I was looking at things wrong or hadn't reached a level in my own practice to be able to answer. Gradually I was mostly correct in my "guesses," and my understanding and experience of Taiji improved by leaps and bounds.

"A teacher can never truly teach unless he is still learning himself."
~ Rabindranath Tagore

Teaching full time, I quickly gained experience and skill in not only my teaching, but through my practice, I was able to refine the Pushing Hands I'd learned from Master Liang into a more comprehensible and scientific arrangement of the teachings, especially for the drill called Willow. When Master Liang taught Willow, he stressed the soft, yielding, neutralizing aspects. As we got more familiar with the defensive aspects, he began to teach how to attack the lines, the Stance-Line, and the center of gravity. At other times he would show us how to add rooting to the Willow, and how we can gradually add hands and stepping. I organized all these teachings into five levels of Willow. The first two are in my Pushing Hands book. I'm sharing all five of these Willows with you in this 40th anniversary book.

Ray Hayward
6th Generation Yang Style Disciple
Season of the Start of Summer
Year of the Dragon 2024

"A teacher affects eternity; he can never tell where his influence stops."
~ Henry Adams

5 Willows

Willow #1 abridged
"A Willow Bends in the Wind"
From my upcoming book *From the Most Soft and Yielding, Taiji Pushing Hands Principles and Practice*, Copyright 2024

"If you want to study pushing hands, begin by investing in loss."
~ Professor Zheng Manqing

The first basic drill, Willow, is by far the most important. Its full name is "The Willow Bends in the Wind" but is usually referred to as "Willow." It is the first drill Master T.T. Liang taught, it is revisited again through the pushing hands curriculum, and it is the last drill taught as a foundation for freestyle Pushing Hands. There is no better exercise for learning and practicing the purely defensive principles. Sometimes we get the best first.

Although it is one of the best methods for learning how to yield, initially it is the hardest because it puts defenders in their most vulnerable position: dealing with attacks by someone in their personal space. This proximity can cause anxiety and increase tension; however, through the study and practice of the Willow exercise, you can learn an array of methods for neutralizing pushing attacks. Willow will teach you the true meaning of balance and unbalance.

In traditional martial arts training, new students are required to endure brutal training methods. My Northern 7-Star Praying Mantis teacher, the late Sifu Lo Man-biu, asked me in my first class if I was ready to "eat bitterness" (chi ku). When I answered yes, he put me in a deep horse stance and told me to hold that for 20 minutes. It was agony! When I stood up my legs were jelly. (If 20 minutes sound short, I suggest you try 5 minutes with a kitchen timer!) He then had me shift from horse stances to bow stances, each for twenty minutes. When it was over, I felt like I did not own my own legs.

My grand teacher, Professor Zheng Manqing, used intelligence and softness to make the bitterness a little easier to understand and endure. He called it "investing in loss." Invest in constant training, lonely hours, defeats, and getting pushed around. At some point you will make gains and be able to take dividends from your investments.

"When a thousand pounds falls on nothing it is useless."
~Yang family teaching

When Master Liang first taught me Willow, he gave the following instructions:

- Don't be afraid to lose: it's an essential part of your development
- Learn how to yield
- Do not begin the study of pushing hands learning to attack
- Unlearn the use of force against force
- Learn to prevent your partner's energy from affecting your balance
- Remember that small loss brings small gain; big loss brings big gain

Master Liang said, "When someone pushes you, you don't resist. Don't be like bulls fighting: yield! If you cannot yield, then let them push you over. Don't resist. Gradually, you will be able to neutralize all your partner's attacks."

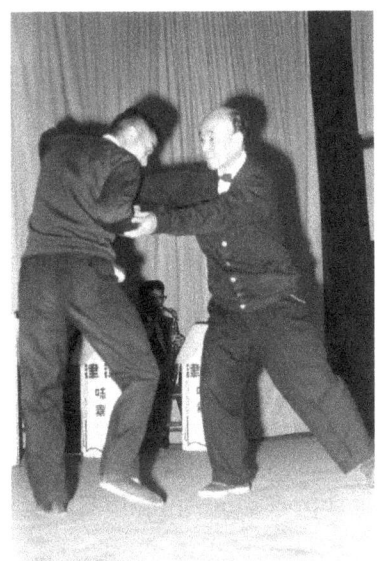

"Fall down seven times, stand up eight."
~ Japanese proverb

Master Liang also said, "The Willow ... exercise is most important: this I must stress. Willow trains the yin and yang to be in coordination. When you push me, I go back, and you come forward. When I push you, I come forward, and you go back. Neutralizing is pushing hands way. You must go back as far as possible and make your body soft, sensitive, and alert."

Additionally, "For beginners, they must learn not to take the initiative. They must learn to lose. Beginners must follow, but mostly they don't want to do it that way." That is, they don't want to follow. But learning to lose by simply giving in will make us soft and teach us how to divert the energy of a push or an attack away from us while remaining lithe as a willow.

The Classics say, "From the most soft and yielding, you will arrive at the most powerful and unyielding." Being soft and studying loss, we will discover what attacks need to be defended. Master William C.C. Chen once told me, "You only need to neutralize people stronger than you. If you are doing pushing hands with a three-year-old, do you need to neutralize them?"

Practicing Willow, you'll become like a Daruma doll with the round bottom that always returns upright. Gradually you'll know which pushes you need to get out of the way of, which ones you can jam or shut in, which ones you can absorb or neutralize, which ones you can intercept, and which ones you can attack.

"I have yet to know of the first person who attained great success without having met and mastered great difficulties, in the form of temporary defeat. Every time a person rises from defeat, they become mentally and spiritually stronger. Thus, in time, one may actually find oneself -their true, inner self- through temporary defeat."
~ Andrew Carnegie

Most martial arts training begins by teaching you to win or conquer your opponent right away. Taiji, however, uses the Taoist concept of opposites: if you want to learn to win, study how to lose. If you want to learn to attack, study how to defend. If you want to learn hardness, study how to be soft. I teach the invest in loss lesson from Master Liang, but I call it "invest in change." From this vulnerable beginning, gradually you'll move toward the perfect defense.

Let me say a quick word about shoes. I suggest getting a good pair of sneakers. Ones that have inner support and a medium tread and provide traction, support, and grip. Taiji slippers and kung-fu booties look cool but can't handle the intensity of real training.

How to begin Willow #1

All the fixed step drills and methods start with the "bow stance" from your Solo Form using the same measurements.

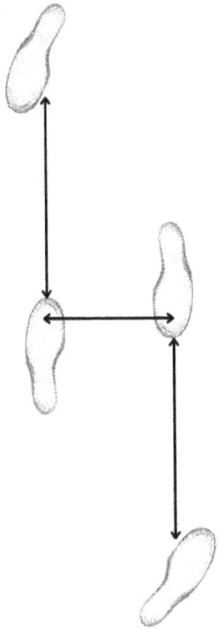

- The partners face each other with either their right or left foot forward
- The balls of your front feet should be in line, across from each other
- The ball of your front foot should line up with the ball of their rear foot

Know the three basic rules for pushing and three basic rules for defending

Defending Side's Rules
1. No resisting
2. No hands or arms
3. No stepping

The first rule, "no resisting," means I should give way and let the pushes move me, or I turn and bend, so the pushes' energy passes by me.
As defenders, we are learning to be soft and yielding. Think of a matador who provokes the bull, and just as the bull is about to attack, the matador pivots and the bull rushes past him. The Taoist concept of wu wei can be translated as "noninterference." The defender does not interfere with or get in the way of incoming energy; they let it pass.

"Embrace uncertainty." ~ Philip Carr-Gomm

When you are touched, you need to un-train the natural reaction of stiffening up, resisting, or pushing against. Later, when you are relaxed and have developed a root, you will learn the correct way and the proper time to root and resist a push. As Master Liang told us, "If you use force against force, you can improve, but gradually, you'll stay there. You cannot reach a high level." When two unyielding people push at the same time, it is force against force, and the stronger person will win. When the founder of Yang Style Taiji, Yang Luchan, first taught publicly, he called his style "cotton fist" or "neutralizing fist," referring to its softness and ability to yield. Think of Muhammed Ali slipping, dodging, or eluding punches.

Trust that a shorter, higher stance, even though it feels too close or more vulnerable, offers a larger turning radius and greater range of motion and will allow for more bend in your knees and greater flexibility in your body.

The second rule, "no hands," means that I cannot use my hands or arms to help me in my defense when neutralizing. Typically, beginners rely on their hands and arms instead of using their whole body. Only with training, when I have learned to unify my body and am relaxed, can I use my hands and arms in conjunction with my whole body for defense.

The third rule, "no stepping," is so that I will learn how to use my waist, my shift, and my relaxation to defend. Stepping is taught in the Dalu, Sanshou, and freestyle pushing hands. Merely stepping out of the way of the push, although a legitimate defense, creates the problem of having to get back in range to counterattack. Stepping back also puts me in an opponent's kicking range. But most importantly for learning Willow #1, stepping back is ill-equipped to teach me how to defend when I have no room to step, like in the corner of a boxing ring or a phone booth. Fixed step is just a training method to help you develop softness. It's not how you use Taiji. Ultimately, you will need to step and move to be effective in your defense.

As you gain skill with softness, you can then deepen your awareness by closing your eyes when you are on the defending side of Willow. And not only Willow, but every basic drill can be taken to the next level by simply closing your eyes and going by touch and feel.

"In this writer's opinion, the basis of all achievement in Tai-Chi Chuan is the fixed-step Push-hands so his advice to the reader is to spend as much time as possible practicing, observing and studying this method."
~ Chen Yanling

Pushing Side's Rules
1. No hit-pushes

2. No boring/sleepy pushes
3. No scratching

As the pusher, we want to learn the correct way to attack our partner's balance, but at this stage, pushing is not for our benefit; it is mostly for the benefit of our partner to help them develop their defenses. That is why the first rule, "no hit-pushes," cuts down on tension and anxiety experienced by the defender. If you are hit as you are pushed, especially in the beginning, you will become tense and fearful. The attacker should first touch softly and then push.

When you are pushing, think of yourself as a coach or trainer. Willow #1 is focused on the defender's side. You are not learning Taiji offense or attack yet.

The second rule, "no boring/sleepy pushes," comes from having had partners who were not present or focused when they pushed me and neglected to feel my body. As the pusher, I need to pay attention to my partner, feeling where they are loose and soft and pushing them where they are stiff or stuck.

The third rule, "no scratching," comes from the years of seeing people leave class with claw marks on their wrists and necks or torn clothes. This is far from the method we want to develop.

Professor Zheng Manqing taught that the body possessed three treasures: 1) the bottom of the weighted foot, 2) the navel, 3) the top of the head. A defensive strategy for Willow #1 is to try to align or balance these three treasures. An offensive strategy is to try to move one or two of these treasures so that their balance is destroyed. If you think of the three treasures as three boxes stacked up, the attacker is trying to shift the boxes, so the stack falls while the defender is trying to shuffle the boxes, so they remain stacked.

Once you start practicing Willow and become familiar with the degree of movement needed to defend, you will be able to refine your technique by what I call active and passive Willow. In active Willow, I move myself. In passive Willow, my partner moves me, and I am like a heavy chain or sack of potatoes. When do I change from active to passive? When my partner's pushes are affecting my balance, I need to move myself. When my partner's pushes don't affect my balance, I become like a sack of potatoes. Experiment with when and where to move yourself, and when and where to let your partner move you. With experience, you will be able to effect the delightful combination of both!

Acquiring Five Skills

Willow is designed to teach you five skills that form the foundation for all defensive skills. These are turning, bending, shifting, sinking, and circling. These five skills may be used singly or combined to make you soft, slippery, and evasive.

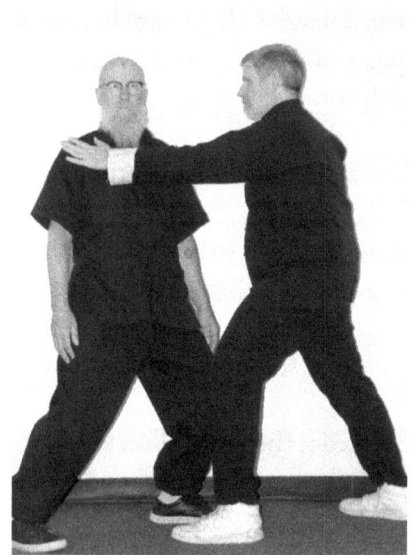

1. Turning: Move your waist and navel from corner to corner, side to side. Or move your waist to one direction, then more in that same direction.

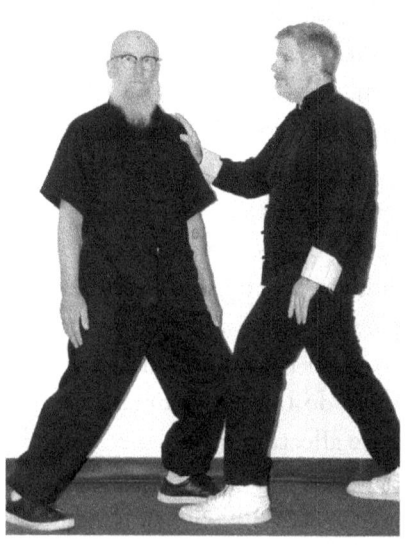
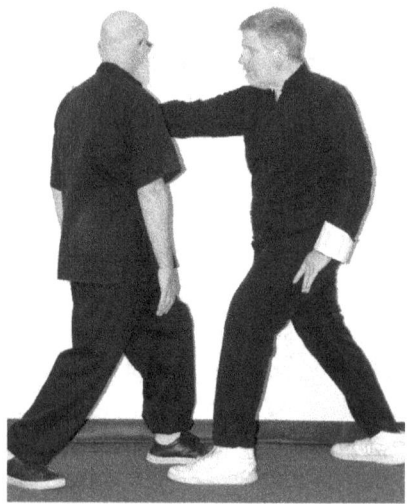

2. Bending: Bend your torso backward, forward, right, or left. Counterbalance gravity using your whole body and stance, not your lower back. For example, if your shoulders are leaning back, let your knees move forward. If your hips are pushed to the right, let your shoulders lean to the left.

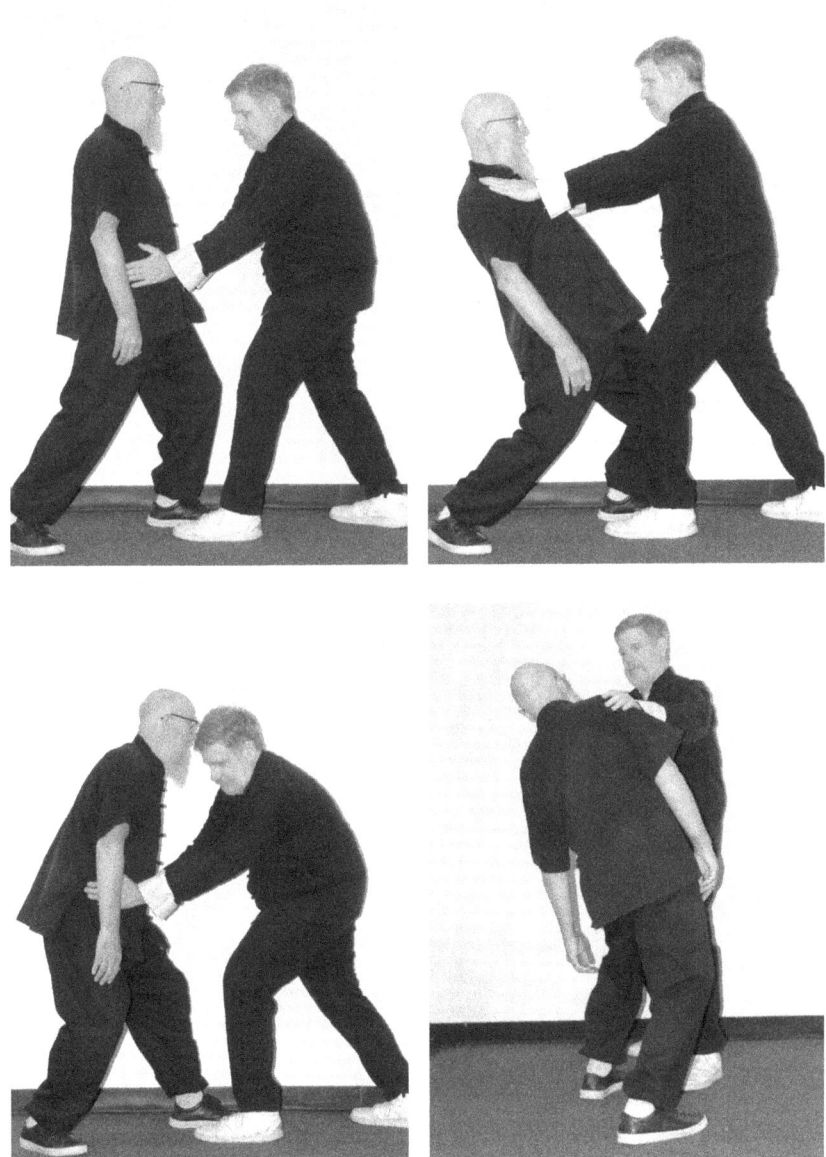

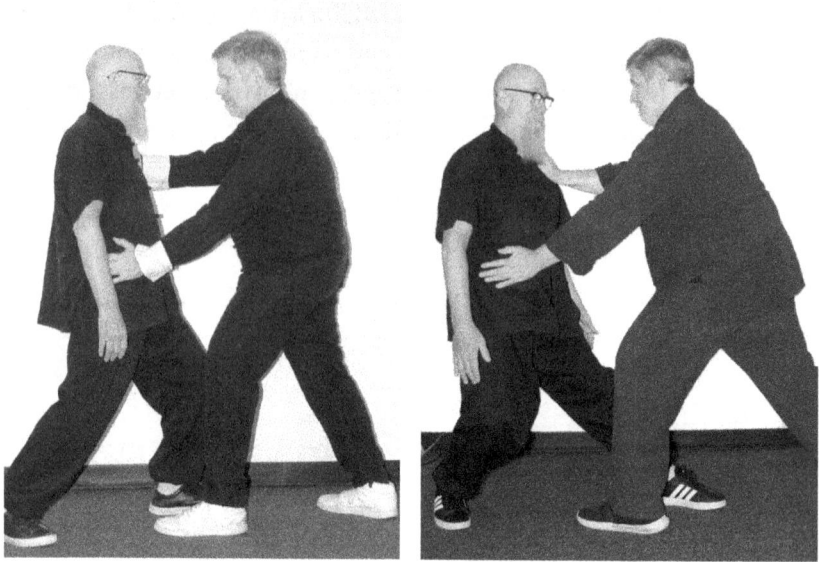

3. Shifting: Push off your front leg to transfer weight to your back leg. Push off your back leg to transfer weight to your front leg. Use your right leg to transfer to the left, and vice versa.

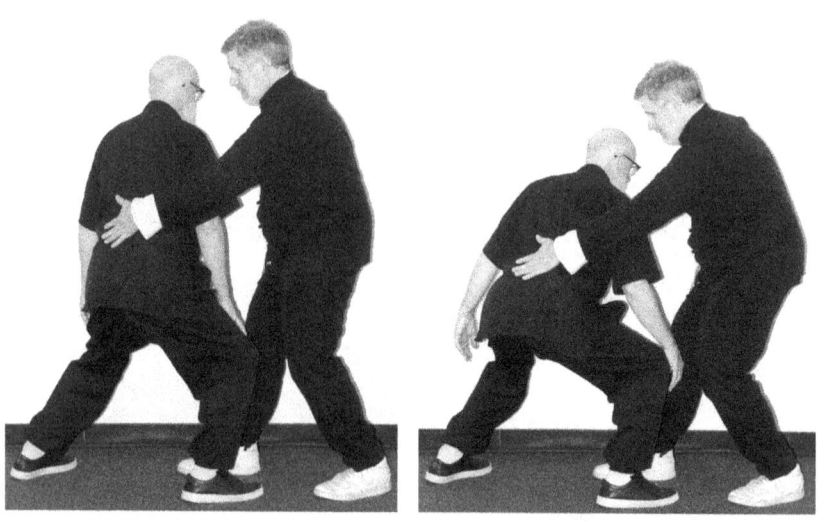

4. Sinking: Relax, drop, soften, sink into your stance and lower your body. Sinking is a good way to catch your balance or to check or stop momentum.

5. Circling: Move a single body part or the whole body in a half or full circle when you have exhausted your ability to turn, bend, shift, or sink.

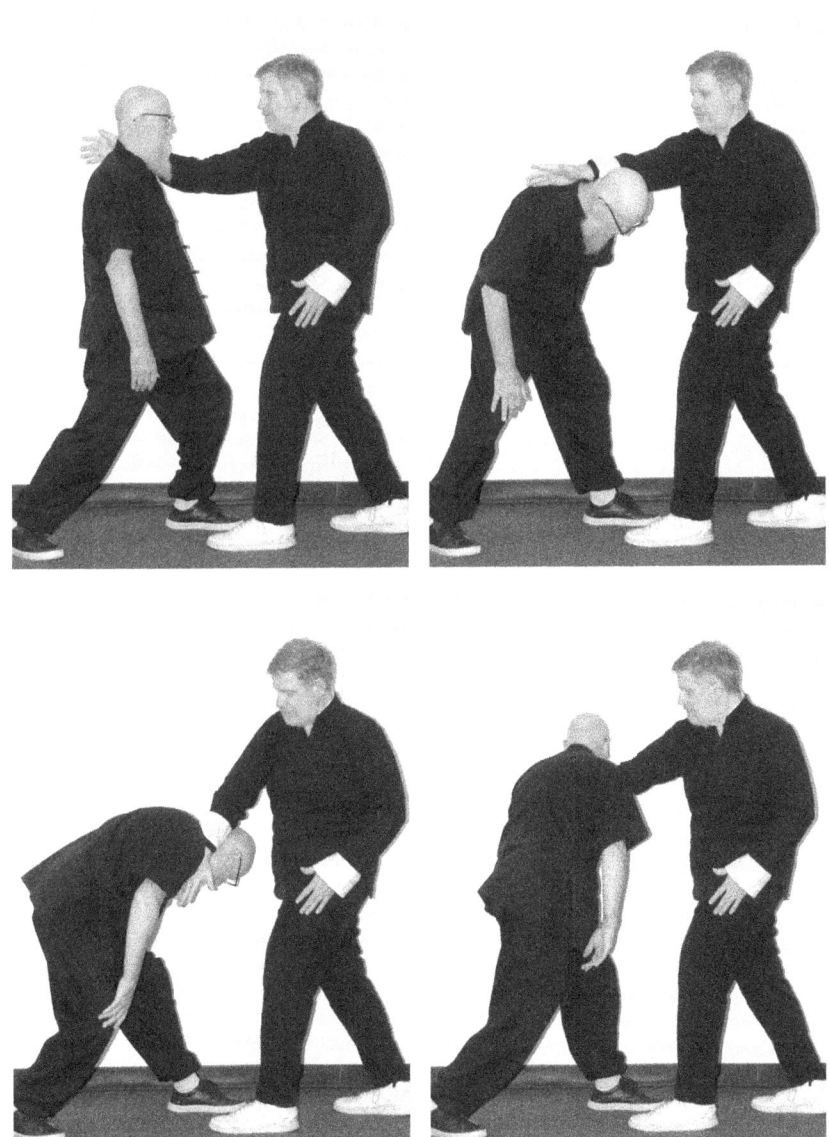

Drill

Stand face to face in a bow stance. Use a timer set for two minutes and have one partner be pushed for two minutes with left foot forward, then another two minutes with the right foot forward. Switch roles. The defender will now push for two minutes with their left foot forward and two minutes with their right foot forward. This constitutes one "round."

If you are the pusher, be deliberate in your pushes and try to unbalance your partner by giving pushes that require them to turn, bend, shift, sink, and circle. Likewise, as defender, try to stay balanced by turning, bending, shifting, sinking, and circling.

This can be repeated as much as you like, or you may go on to other drills and methods. You could do one round of the Willow, switch to another drill or method, return to another round of the Willow, then another method, continually checking your foundation of softness, relaxation, and sensitivity.

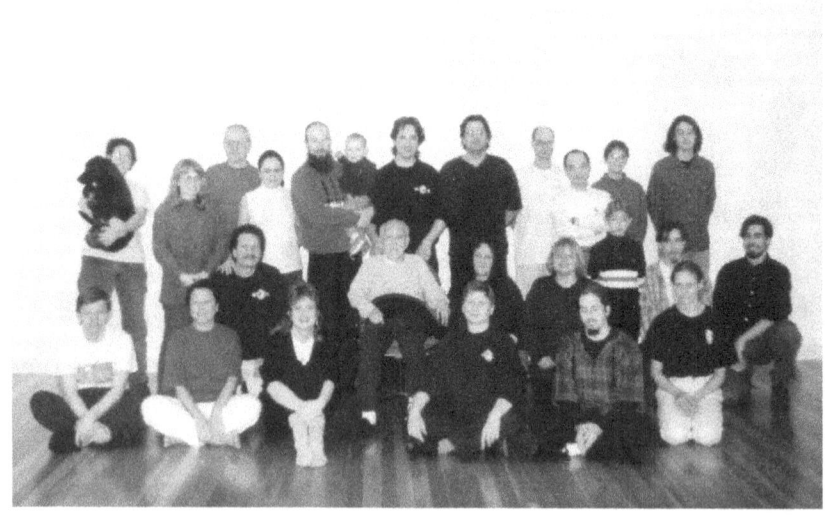

Willow #2 abridged
"Find the Line"

From my upcoming book *From the Most Soft and Yielding, Taiji Pushing Hands Principles and Practices* Copyright 2024

In Willow #1, the pushing or attacking side is like a coach, trainer, or helper: they attack fear, tension, inflexibility, and anticipation. The pusher helps the defender train their neutralizing skills, using their attacks to help their partner develop the softness, flexibility, and evasiveness required in Taiji defense.

In Willow #2, that all changes. The training is now for the pushing side. Here is where you learn the Taiji art of attacking. To offset our opponent's balance or cause internal damage, the pusher's attacks focus on three main places:

+ Stance-Line
+ Centerline
+ Center of gravity

When you begin pushing, you first must detect whether your partner is stiff and tense or soft and loose. If they are hard or tense, they tie up themselves, and everywhere you touch will lead you to the Stance-Line, centerline, and center of gravity. If your partner is soft or loose, you must tie them up with three pieces of rope: 1) centerline, 2) center of gravity, 3) stance-line, and then you can push.

An analogy for this difference is that of lifting or moving an iron bar versus a chain. An iron bar is a metaphor for a stiff, tense, hard, substantial opponent. Anywhere you touch or move the iron bar affects the whole bar. An iron chain is a metaphor for a soft, relaxed, supple, insubstantial opponent. Only the place you touch is affected. If your partner is loose, you will have to package them up like a chain to move them. For pushing hands, you either have to make them tense or learn the three places to attack to move them.

To do Willow #2 drill correctly, the defender simply uses their Willow #1 skills. The attacker uses the three methods of Taiji issuing energy: on a plane, in a line, and at a point. These must be drilled separately so that when the time comes in Willow #2 to issue one of these three energies, you use your whole body to push—not just your arms and hands.

The Yang's family training manual states that when we begin learning to attack, we must start with a compass, and there are three different compasses to look at:

- The first compass is horizontal to the ground as if your opponent is standing on a compass. This helps us learn the Stance-Lines.

- The second compass is vertical with the head being North and the feet being South. This helps us learn the centerline.

- The third compass is also vertical, but with the front of their body being West (or East) and their back being East (or West). This helps us learn the center of gravity.

1. Stance-Line

"Each single part of the body has both a substantial and an insubstantial aspect at any given time."
~ Taiji Classics

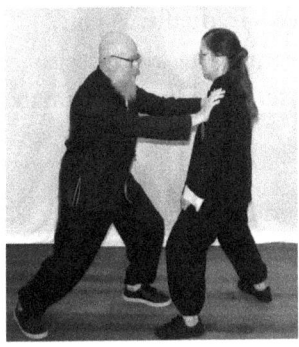 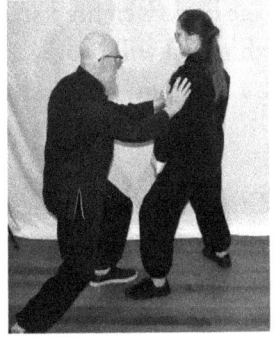 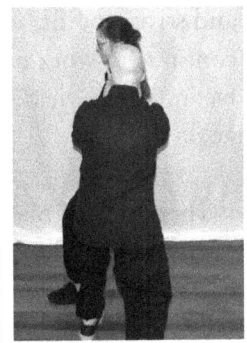

One simple exercise is to have your partner stand in a bow stance, with 70 to 80% of their weight on the front foot, and imagine they are standing on a compass. Give them light pushes in each of the eight directions, while you move from North to South, changing your angle, but keeping your partner in place, and pushing from northeast to southwest, etc. As you go around the compass points, you will naturally feel the strong and weak points of their stance as well as some neutral aspects.

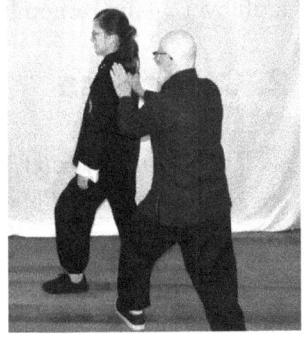

Do both legs, then have them shift back so that 70 to 80% of their weight is now on their back foot. Again, imagine they are standing on a compass or mark the lines on the floor, then go around pushing, letting your hands feel and catalogue the weak

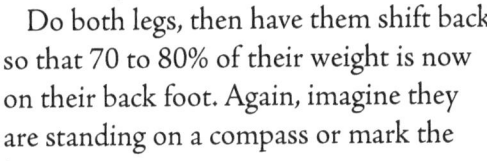

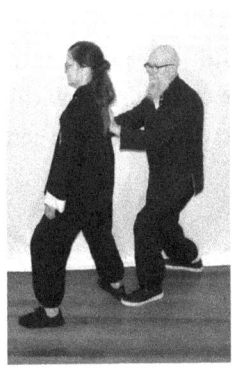 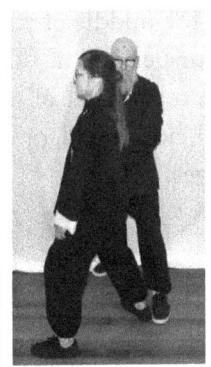 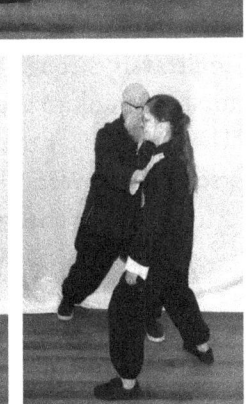

and strong points of the back-weighted stance. Gradually, as you continue to work on this, you will progress from seeing the lines to feeling them, yielding a much quicker response, which is the ultimate goal.

Then switch roles. Stand in a bow stance and have your partner push you in eight directions. You begin to feel in your own body where your stances are naturally strong, where your stances are naturally weak, and those in between. Then shift your weight back and do it all over again, remembering to do both legs.

2. Centerline

"If you gain the center, you will win. If you lose the center, you will lose. This is a fixed principle."
~ Yang Shaohou

After the stance-line, I teach the centerline. Master Choi always taught the centerline first, and I agree it's the most important for martial arts; however, for pushing hands, the stance-line is the most important. Pushing-hands is but one aspect of Taiji as a martial art and focuses on off-balancing more than on striking.

The centerline is an invisible line starting at the top of your head, the crown chakra, and travels through the middle of your torso or trunk to your perineum. Think of your body as a cylinder. The centerline is the very center of the cylinder. Now the cylinder itself may be vertical, horizontal, or diagonal, but the centerline of the cylinder never changes.

"The whole goal of martial arts is to protect your centerline and control the opponent's centerline."
~ Wang Hsiang-chai

People sometimes confuse the plumb line with the centerline. The plumb line is an invisible line of gravity passing downward through the torso and stance. The plumb line is vertical whether your torso is vertical, horizontal, or diagonal; whereas the centerline is consistent with the angle of the torso and will move and change as the torso moves and changes from vertical to horizontal to any other direction.

If a force goes directly to the center of the cylinder, the whole cylinder will be affected. If the force misses the center of the cylinder, the cylinder will naturally turn, and the power of the push will be diminished. Or as in neutralizing, the person starts to turn their waist, which rotates the cylinder and turns the attack off their centerline.

In Willow #1, I avoid pushing my partner's centerline, so they will learn to neutralize by turning. In Willow #2, I don't want my opponent to turn, which will deflect my push; rather, I want to keep their torso stationary, so I aim all my pushes at their center, straight through, to affect the cylinder, and consequently their torso, making it difficult for them to maintain balance.

3. Center of Gravity

"Sometimes this means I catch your center of gravity, just the middle of your body. The shoulders are too high, the hips are too low."
~ Master T.T. Liang

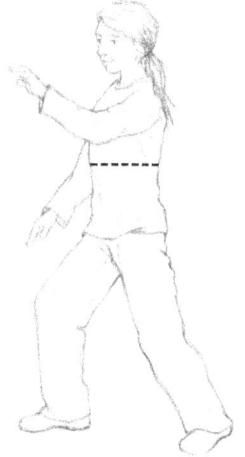

The third aspect is the center of gravity, which is the halfway point between the top and bottom of a vertical cylinder (i.e. your torso). Master Liang would say you have to know where the center of gravity is. The shoulders are above the center, and the hips are below, so you must push the middle, around the solar plexus, which is also the location of the liver, kidneys, spleen, and the solar plexus itself (and is why keeping our elbows down protects us from strikes to this vulnerable area).

Say, for example, a cylinder is suspended in space. If you push near the top, it will start spinning backward. If you push near the bottom, it will start spinning forward. If you push the middle of the cylinder, the whole cylinder moves backward. Imagining this cylinder will greatly improve your pushing technique.

If your hands are above the center of gravity, your pushes and strikes must go slightly downward to offset that area. (This is why Xingyi teaches to punch slightly downward.) If your hands are below the center of gravity, your pushes and strikes must go slightly upward to offset that area. If your hands are center of gravity height, push horizontally.

Establish your practice strategy

"First in the mind, then in the body."
~ Taiji Classics

At this point I've given you a lot of information. These are the principles, classics, and secret techniques all explained simply and clearly. Now you have a lot of work to do! There is a great difference between intellectually understanding how these techniques work and being able to execute them. Master Choi would say, "One hour in the mind needs 100 hours of practice to get it into the body."

You must be patient and adhere to a practice strategy to hone your ability to attack the stance-line, centerline, and center of gravity simultaneously. What made the Yang family so good was that they began training as young children and had many years to perfect their attacks. Most of us don't begin training in our youth, so I have devised a strategy to help you, distilled from my 30 years of practice and teaching.

For pushing, begin by attacking your opponent's Stance-Lines. Concentrate on attacking only one or two lines each time it's your

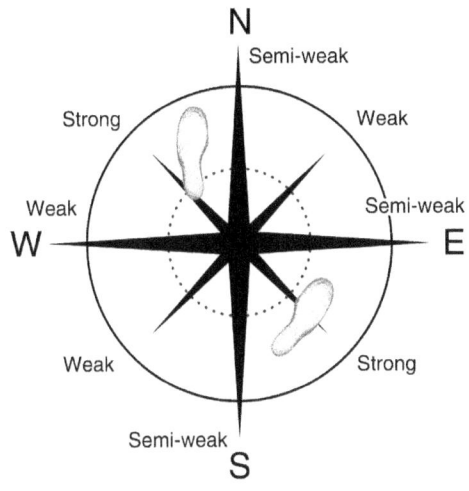

turn to push. Think of the eight directions of the compass on the floor, use your eyes to locate the weak points and directions of your partner's stances. Avoid the two directions where their feet are positioned, which would go directly into their root or leg. Gradually you will be able to feel the weak directions even as your partner moves and adapts to your pushes.

Then concentrate only on your partner's centerline. Make sure all your pushes go directly through the very center of their torso, no matter the direction or angle of their body. You'll know when you're pushing off the centerline because they'll either turn or spin, or you'll feel your pushing power weakening. When you're on the centerline, you'll feel it, even as it's changing, but you will still be able to continue pushing straight through it.

Finally, concentrate only on your partner's center of gravity. Do not push above or below their solar plexus. Get your hands on the very midpoint of their torso and push. If your hands aren't on the midpoint, don't push. Later, when you are able to locate the center of gravity, push upwards if you are below the center of gravity, and slightly downwards if you are above their center of gravity.

The defending side in Willow #2 needs to be patient and think of themselves as a training partner or coach. If you have a hard time staying in your stance and are constantly getting pushed out, this is really good! That means your partner is learning how to attack your Stance-Line, centerline, and center of gravity. I know it can be frustrating but just hang in there and make sure you get your turn as well. Remember not to resist, use your arms, or step away—and don't worry: in Willow #3 I'll teach you how to defend these Willow #2 attacks.

Master Liang's formula for attacking the line

"You must find the line, exactly on the line, then push with the whole body."
~ Master T. T. Liang

Although Master Liang would sometimes call all three aspects "the line," he really meant the line or direction of your attacking energy, and he taught a simple formula to practice and acquire these attacking skills.

1. Find the line.
You are doing that right now by learning to locate the Stance-Lines, centerline, and center of gravity. First you have to understand the concepts. Next you need some practical knowledge and demonstrations of where they are. Then you need to learn to find those lines and weak points in your opponent's body and stances, as well in your own body and stances. Understanding why and how these all work is the essential first step to increasing your pushing skill.

2. Push the line.
Once you know where you are going to push, you have to know how to push, utilizing one of the three ways of issuing Taiji energy: 1) on a plane or arc, 2) in a straight line, 3) at a single point. Long power pushes teach us how to issue energy on a plane or an arc; short-power advanced drills teach us how to issue energy at a single point.

Either way, don't push with just your hands or arms. If you do, your power comes from above your partner's center of gravity making it difficult to lift them. If you push with your legs, your power comes from below their center of gravity, and you can easily lift them. Whole body power can change the direction, but arms usually only push in one direction. Furthermore, your arms are not as strong as your whole body. When the opportunity comes to attack the line, you must do it in Taiji fashion, which is whole body power–that is, upper and lower parts coordinated, starting together/stopping together.

3. Change the line.

When you are pushing and it isn't working, you can change to a new line or direction. This can be done in two ways. One way is to use the same hand but change the direction of your push. For example, if you're pushing north, you can start to push northeast. The other way is to use the other hand to push a new line or direction.

Sometimes when your partner defends one of your arms, they make an opening for your other arm. If they can neutralize one of your hands and arms, you can issue through the other one. This is a simple but effective technique. You push with one arm or hand, and if that is neutralized, use the other hand and push a different line.

This is why Professor Zheng said beginners can push with two hands, but advanced people should push with one hand. If you always push with two hands, and they neutralize, your power will be ineffective.

4. Follow the line

"The power of the turbulent flow is difficult to resist.
Coming to a high place, it swells and fills the place up.
Meeting a hollow it dives downward.
There are troughs and crests un the waves.
There is no opening into which it does not enter."
~ Secrets of the Eight Postures Classic

Of course, your partner is going to try to neutralize your attacks, and as they willow, i.e. shift, bend, turn, etc. you must follow them, continually attacking or seeking to attack. Once you are on their centerline or center of gravity, you must stick with it, no matter where they move — keep on it, following and pushing. When they try to neutralize your push or hide their center, become like a heat-seeking missile by sticking and adhering to them. Only when they are stuck with the weak part of their stance open and their centerline and center of gravity in your sights, issue your power and push them away. As Master Liang always told us, "Don't push blindly."

5. Set up the line.

Once you are comfortable issuing energy through just one arm or hand, Willow #2 becomes like a chess game, where you plan your attacks, using your first push as a set up. For example, you can gently push with one arm, maneuvering them to open their Stance-Line. When they turn or move, you can push through their centerline and center of gravity with the other hand.

There is a Chinese saying, "Signal west and attack east." You push with one hand, they move and neutralize, but you have set them up for the real attack, which is your other hand. There are many ways to set up a line. You can also think about pulling a shoulder forward as a set-up just as you would push a shoulder backward to make an opening.

6. Control the line.

Sometimes Master Liang would use energy with one hand or arm and literally hold you in place while he pushed with the other hand. You can't use too much energy when you control because they can use it against you to withdraw-attack. In some situations, your partner is in the perfect position for your attack with their Stance-Line open, their centerline controlled, and you knowing whether you are above, on, or below their center of gravity. Now you control them, seize them, or hold them in place, so you can execute your attack. To achieve this, you have to be able to separate your arms into insubstantial and substantial and have a degree of control over your hard and soft so that each arm expresses different energies: i.e. one controls, and one attacks.

7. Ti Fang

Ti Fang, also known as "lift-let go" or "withdraw and push" or "push-pull," is one of the five advanced drills I learned from Master Liang. Ti Fang makes your opponent resist and float, which is the opposite of the Taiji foundation of relax and sink. Think of someone on a diving board. When they jump and are springing up, there is a point when they stop rising but haven't started descending. They are at zero gravity. If something were to push them at that moment, they would not be able to resist or root and would go far away. The "Ti" in Ti Fang is to bring your opponent to zero-gravity before pushing.

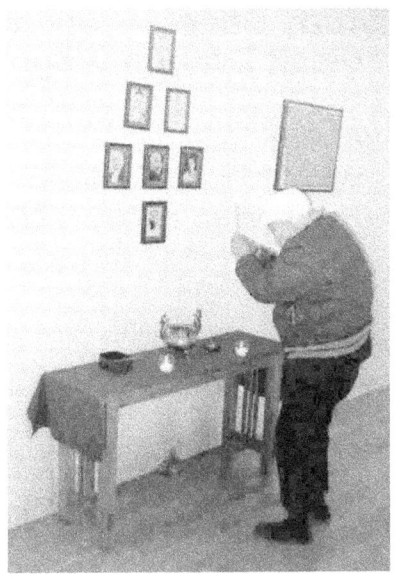

When your partner resists you, or you make them resist you, you withdraw to make them lose balance or "fall up." When they lose balance, they tense up and become top-heavy, which automatically binds together the centerline and center gravity and makes all directions of their stance weak. That's when you do the Fang, which literally means to "release a bird," you push or release them.

Master Liang always used Ti Fang for stiff, strong, resisting opponents. When you push to open a line or maneuver your partner into a defective position, sometimes you will meet resistance, either on purpose or not. Instead of forcing your way through, simply withdraw to break their root, make them fall up, then push.

As with learning the Stance-Line, centerline, and center of gravity, take these formulas one at a time, and after you learn to apply them singly, start using them together or let circumstances dictate which ones you use. Or use them all! Remember, if your push isn't working, the answer is not to use more tension, force, or power: the answer is to use more knowledge, technique, and your whole body. Push smarter, not harder!

Study Sheet — Willow #3
"Black Dragon Wags Its Tail"

Perspective

- Willow #3 is 80% for the defending side. Techniques and ideas on how to protect the Stance-Line, centerline, and center of gravity. To do this, Willow#3 changes the defender rules of Willow#1.

- No resistance becomes rooting, shutting in, and jamming.

- No hands become all manner of techniques from the basic drills, methods, and sticking drills, summed up by calling them all Ward Off.

- No stepping becomes Taiji footwork; light, nimble, balanced, agile, as well as being rooted.

  "Everybody knows how to hit; the skill is in defense."
  ~ Grandmaster Wai-lun Choi

1. Adding arms to Willow #3 to defend the centerline. The arms are to hide and guide.

- Add arms to the basic Willow #1 techniques of turning, bending, shifting, circling, and sinking.

- Use the arms from the basics drill, such as upward split. You have 8 from your basic drills available.

- Reach out and stick, absorb, receive, investigate.

  "Neutralize the opponent's incoming force with outstretched arms."
  ~ Yang Banhou

- Inside the arm, stick closer to the wrist. Outside the arm, stick closer to the elbow. Master Choi's auger idea= coiling or being a corkscrew, moving up or down their arms.

- 3 joints of the arm are for different size changes. Wrists for small changes, elbows for medium changes, and shoulders for biggest changes.

- 5 Elements of Sticking, Adhere, Join, Stick, Follow, No Resistance/No Letting Go.

- Coil, drill, snake, and roll.

- The two most useful techniques, Roll Back and Split.

- Simple strategy-if they push with two hands, either Split or Roll Back. If they push with one hand, either stick or coil.

- Add arms to body movements, don't substitute arms for whole body technique!

  "…one will have reached the stage in which one can yield everywhere at the opponent's slightest pressure and adhere to his slightest retreat."
  ~ Master T.T. Liang

2. Adding stepping to Willow#3 to defend the Stance-Line. Two boats passing in the water, the size of the wake is the size of your step.

- Only step as much as you need.
- Stance height change/Three kinds of stances.
- Ankles and 9 Joint Unity.
- Shuffle/stealing/follow step.
- Angle change.
- Change step.
- Toe to Toe.
- 4 directions stepping/5 directions stepping.
- Circle walk.
- Simple strategy- more stepping use less hands and rooting, less stepping use more hands and rooting.

"Therefore, in our movement practice, the most important thing is coordinating steps in pushing-hands."
~ Professor Zheng Manqing

3. Adding rooting to Willow #3 to defend the center of gravity. Never just root.

- Use your root to help your defense.
- Root for a half second to change from split to roll back and roll back to split.
- Jam, or shut in, a push to your center of gravity.
- Use rooting to guide a push into your back leg, then turn.
- Root fast hand attacks.
- Save rooting for need only.
- Root and turn/change/step.

"The most important thing is what? You must have equilibrium! You can just stand there, and no one can push you over. But you don't use it. Just like you have atomic bombs, but don't use them."
~ Master T.T. Liang

*Attack side reminder, you are still pushing the centerline, Stance-Line, and center of gravity.

** Willow #3 is also the basic practice for Sword Sticking/Sensitivity and can be adapted for Taiji Sword fencing.

"For real fighting, you have to get the perfect defense."
~ Grandmaster Wai-lun Choi

Willow #4 — Study Sheet

"There is no opening into which it does not enter…"

Perspective

Willow #4 is 80% for the attacking side. Techniques and ideas on how to attack when they can hide their centerline with their hands, firm their center of gravity with rooting, and close their Stance-Line with footwork. To do this, Willow #4 changes the attacking side's rules of Willow #1. There are two versions to this level: Pushing and Striking. One for sensitivity and one for self-defense.

For Pushing,
- No hit-pushes becomes, short power, finger to palm, ti fang, changes in speed or intensity.
- No boring/sleepy pushes, becomes, bore them, put them to sleep, ambush, trap, fakes, surprises.
- No scratching becomes, the correct time, and way, to use Pull for seizing and off balance.

For Striking,
- No hit-pushes becomes, strikes, short power, finger to palm, ti fang, fakes, scare, hit pushes, feints, surprise attacks.
- No boring/sleepy pushes, becomes, bore them, put them to sleep, ambush, set ups, trap, feints, surprises.
- No scratching becomes, the correct time, and way, to use Pull for attack.
- 3 Forwards, 7 Stars, 8 Ultimates.

1. For hands and arms.
- Push/Pull/ Ti Fang stiff arms.
- Trap, Pin, Manipulate soft arms.
- Develop other energies besides Push: Ward Off, Shoulder, Elbow, Press, Diagonal Flying etc.
- Folding Technique.
- Withdraw-Attack.
- Whoever breaks contact must be struck/pushed.
- Na- Control or Seize.

"After first the contact, you have to chase their hands. We chase their hands, so they don't get free. Then you try to trap their hands."
~ Grandmaster Wai-lun Choi

2. For Stepping.
+ Make them root.
+ Herd them.
+ 7 Stars Step, sweep and tread.

> "There is also use of the foot. The foot techniques are important: sweeping, tripping, and all these techniques. If you sweep me, I lift my foot to neutralize, then step in and push."
> ~ Master T.T. Liang

3. For Rooting.
+ Ti Fang.
+ Angle Change.
+ Fake/Scare.

> "If someone had stiff arms when practicing pushing hands with Professor Zheng, he would pull or push them through their arms."
> ~ Master T.T. Liang

Willow #5 — Study Sheet

"When attacking above, you must not below."

Perspective, both sides may attack or defend or both.

> "Control you, I hit. Don't control you, don't hit."
> ~ Grandmaster Wai-lun Choi

+ Know the difference—Practicing, Training, Sparring, Competition, Fighting, Self-defense, Survival.
+ Professor Zheng's two-man saw analogy.
+ Free Style or Sanshou.
+ Tung Chin, Interpreting Energy.
+ Some Taiji Classics.

"One side attacks, the other side concentrates on listening. Get used to it. When you feel better, then both sides can attack."
~ Grandmaster Wai-lun Choi

6 safe competitions:
- Move feet— try to make your partner move their feet or take a step.
- Uproot— try to lift your partner out of their stance and make both their feet leave the ground.
- Past a line — pick a line or mark and try to get them to move back past that line.
- Into a wall/mattress — make them fall back and lose their stance and balance.
- Out of circle — make them step one or both feet out of a circle.

"Sensitivity and explode power are the essentials."
~ Grandmaster Wai-lun Choi

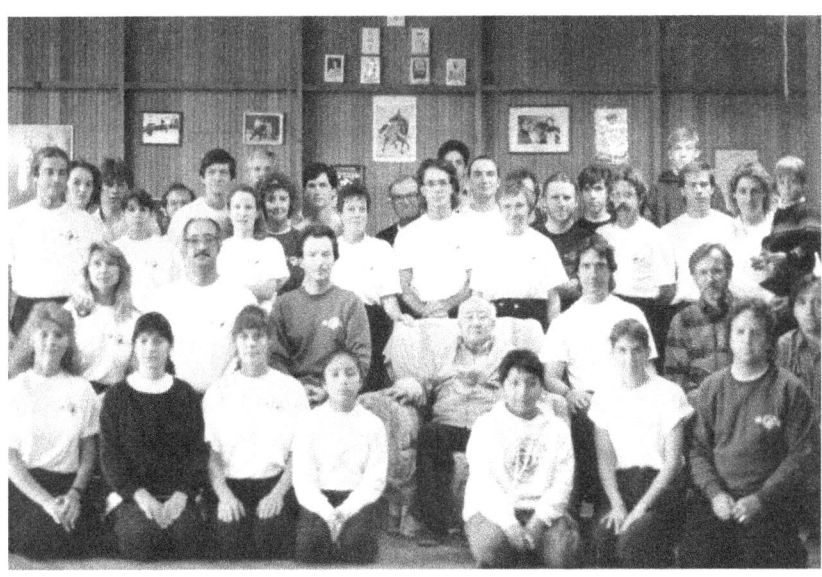

Photo essay.
By Ray Hayward

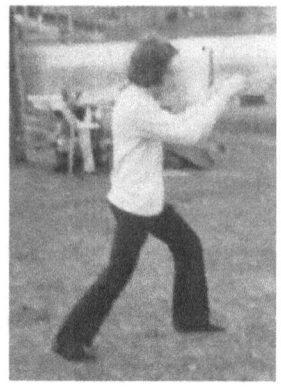

Sifu Ray's first Push photo in Lynnfield Mass..

"Now you know this solo form. Externally it is ok, but internally a lot of things you have to remember. Externally the postures may be correct, but internally quite incorrect. Something may not be quite right. You must presume you have an opponent in front of you. Some energy must be at the top of your head all the time to suspend it. Also, use intrinsic energy, do not be double-weighted – a lot of things. You have to know how to breathe, at what point do you inhale or exhale, what time to push -a lot of things you have to know."
~ Master T.T. Liang (quote about my solo form from 1981)

On Labor Day of 1984, I had a set of photos of my Solo Form taken at East River Flats Park. I wanted to see my Solo Form from the outside and make corrections and refinements. I have taken other sets throughout the years, and my Sword Form a few times as well. This year, 2024, I'm taking another set of photos again for corrections, refinement, and something else, to catalogue and witness what 40 years of learning, practicing, and teaching Taiji has done to my form and my body. Of course it's only the outside you can see, but I can tell you about some of my inner changes. Some of my oldest friends, classmates, and students can address any changes to my personality and temperament. Here is some of what I see from both looking at the outside and knowing myself from the inside.

"Only rebels can get something."
~ Master T.T. Liang

After years of learning, practicing, and teaching, I started to have my own ideas about my form. My experience started to influence how I moved. Studying with Master Liang, he always encouraged me to find my own way, my own Solo Form. He would point out how the Yang's family and their advanced students all did their forms a little bit differently. The sequences were the same, the principles and the classics were the same, but the execution and flavor became personal.

"Do you still have a black and white T.V.?"
~ Grandmaster Wai-lun Choi

When I began to study with Grandmaster Wai-lun Choi, he always taught that I should have my applications fit modern fighting, not the old-fashioned fighting of decades ago. For instance, he told me to adapt the applications for boxing and wrestling, plus Thai Kickboxing leg kicks, which is how most people fight nowadays. Not to teach applications for kung-fu strikes, or Bagua and Taiji attacks. He also encouraged me to investigate sports, health, and breath sciences so I could improve the training methods.

Studying with my two main teachers, I had the wonderful dilemma of having more than one right answer! Both masters, Liang and Choi, had different mechanics for movement, stances, and applications in the Solo Form. For instance, Liang's methods were more for pushing, whereas Choi's were more for punching. I blended Master Liang's "Whole Body as One Unit," which is mostly for pushing, with Master Choi's "9 Joint Harmony," (which I call 9 Joint Unity) mostly for striking.

Master Liang taught that the spine should be plumb erect. Master 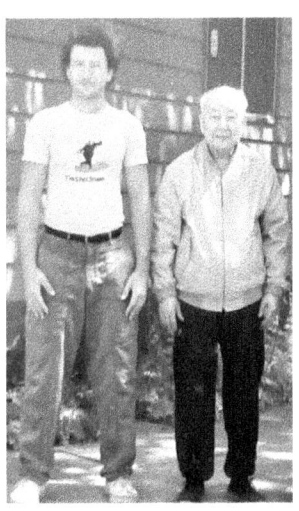 Choi said I should always be aware of the invisible plumbline of gravity going through my body and stance. I call these plumb spine and plumbline. For Liang, the plumbline and the spine were always together. For Choi, the plumbline and the spine were together when the weight was on the back foot, or you were standing up, otherwise the spine was forward of plumb. Over the last twenty years I gradually synthesized both master's methods into my own Solo Form, without violating the classics, the theories, the principles, or my masters' generous teachings.

Plumb Line

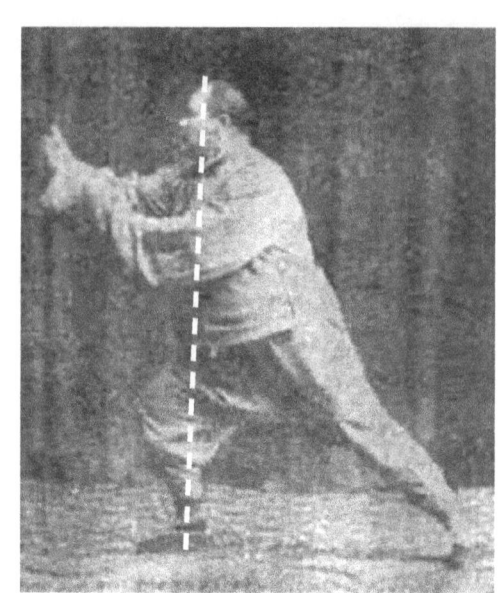
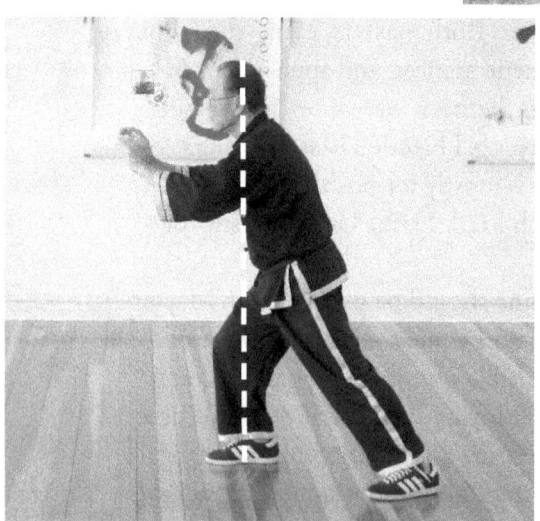
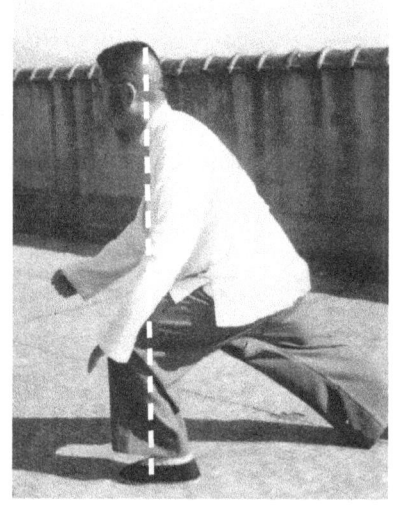

Plumb Spine

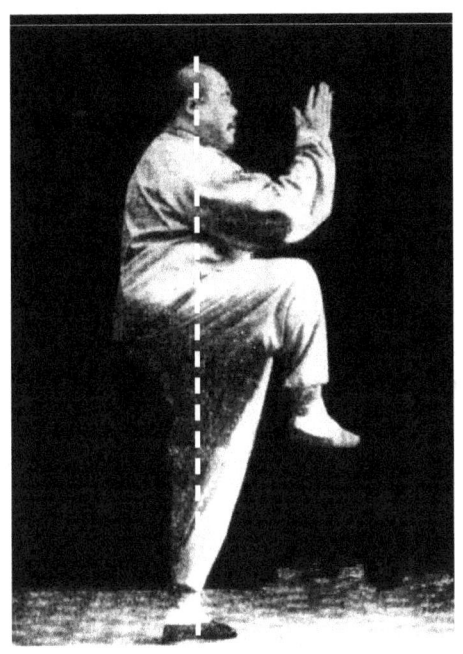

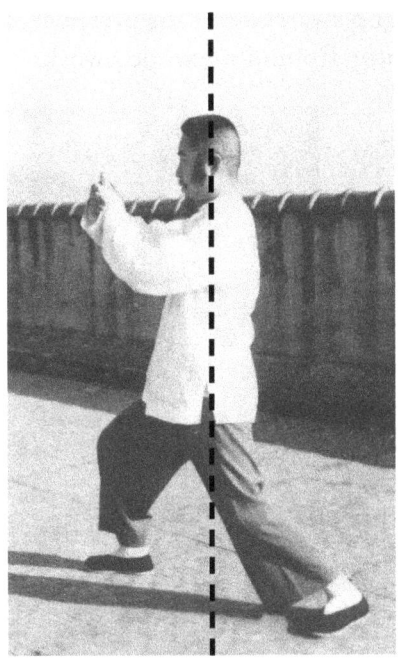

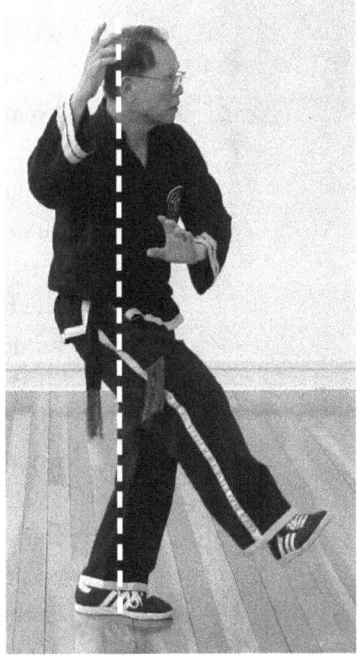

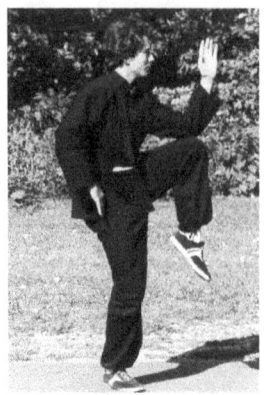

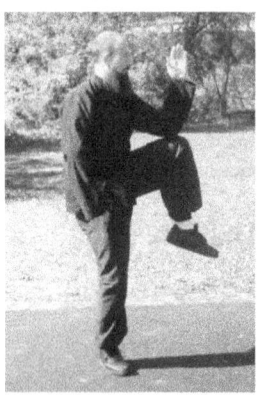

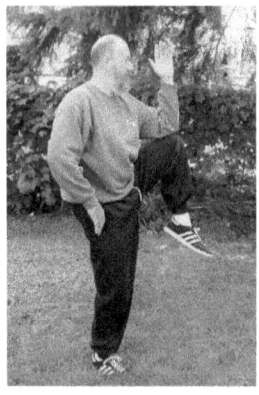

1984- Looking at my postures, you can see that I was working on getting low, strong stances, gaining a root, and strengthening my legs. Master Liang always complimented me on my low stances and agile footwork. I was kicking high for strength and self-defense. I worked a lot on Long Power and every aspect of shifting and transferring weight. The other thing I worked on was getting the heights, measurements, angles, counts, and directions correct. My frame was large to medium. I felt that if I got the externals correct, they would influence my internal and technique as well. Internally I was working on exact breathing patterns to circulate energy and had, and still have, many experiences of the movement of chi, and heat/cold/tingling/rushing sensations throughout my body during the form. I also worked on having the feeling and awareness of the presence of an opponent in front of me while I worked through applications in my mind.

Of the twin foundations of relax and sink, in those early days I was primarily working on sink.

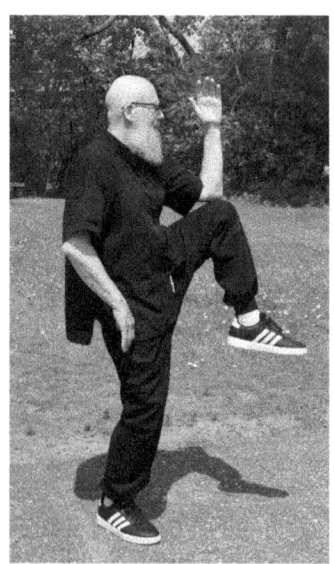

2024- Looking at my postures today, you can see my emphasis is on how the postures feel, as opposed to how they look. I am working on unity, 9 Joint Unity, or whole-body coordination, which leads me to now work mainly on short power. I am not concerned with my spine being plumb, but I am working with the ever-constant plumbline of gravity passing through my body and structure. I'm more forward now, using Master Choi's simple alignment of having my head over a foot. When I'm front weighted, I'm forward having a foot under my head. When I'm back weighted, I am plumb and have my head, hips, and foot in a vertical line.

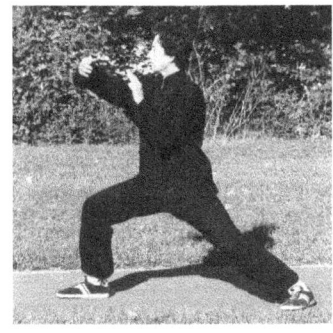

I kick high now for flexibility and range of motion. I am working on "under breathing" and letting my natural breath patterns adjust to what they need. I try not to bother, interfere, or manage my breathing, and let my breath do whatever my Solo Form demands.

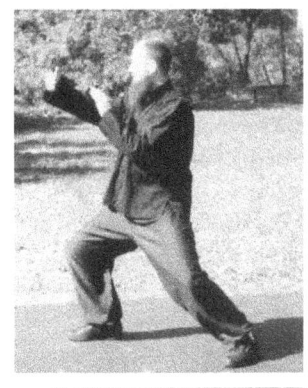

I have three ways I work my Solo Form, slow, flow, and low. The first decades I mostly worked on going slow, taking up to forty minutes to do the solo form and doing the stances as low as I could. Now I mostly work on flow, and that takes me between twenty to twenty-five minutes for a round. I also used to train holding postures for a long time, but now I hold for a much shorter time. My frame is mostly medium, and some small.

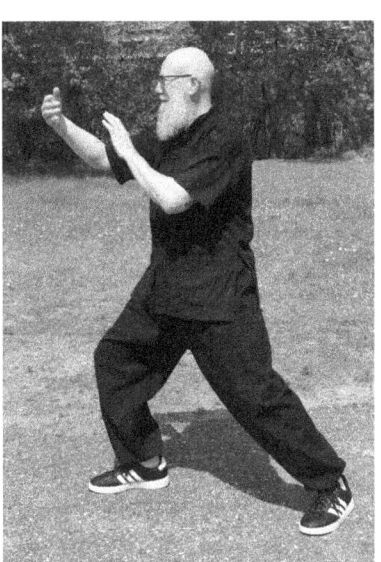

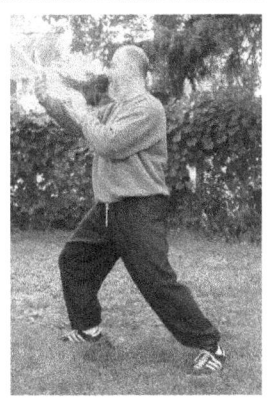

111

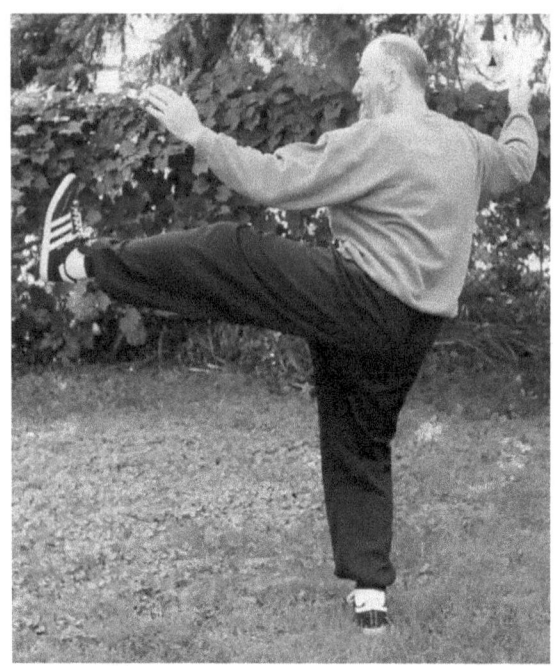

Internally I am working on being natural, and letting my spirit guide my body. Witnessing chi movement as opposed to trying to direct or lead where it goes.

Of the twin foundations of relax and sink, these days I'm primarily working on relax.

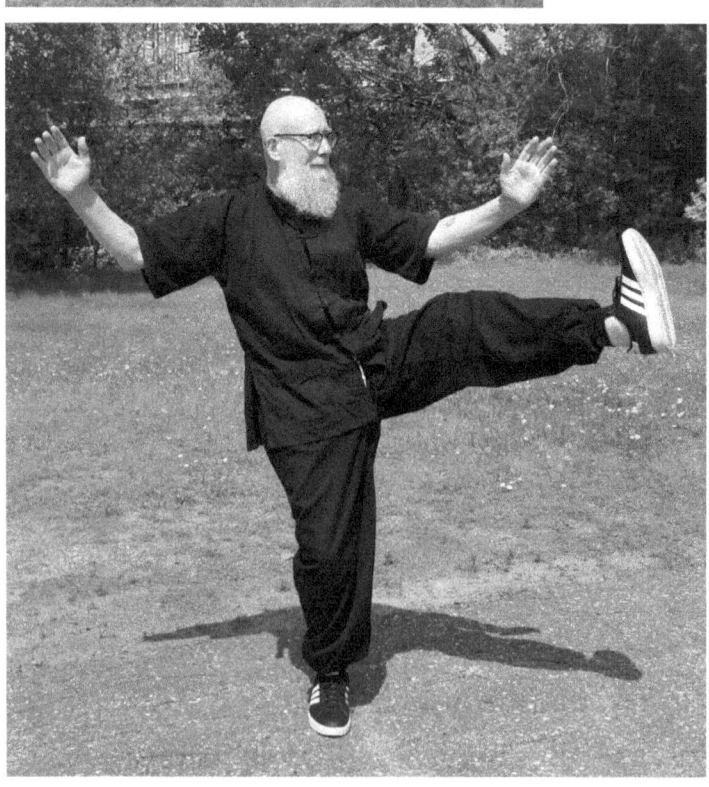

"Raise the Curtain"

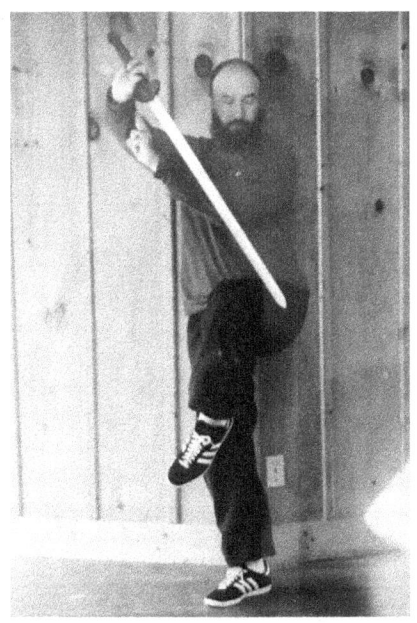
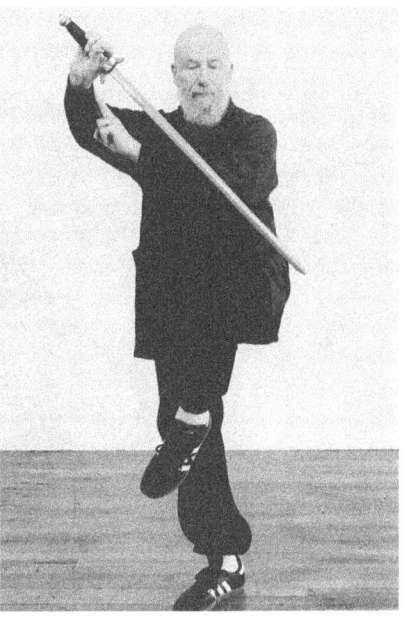
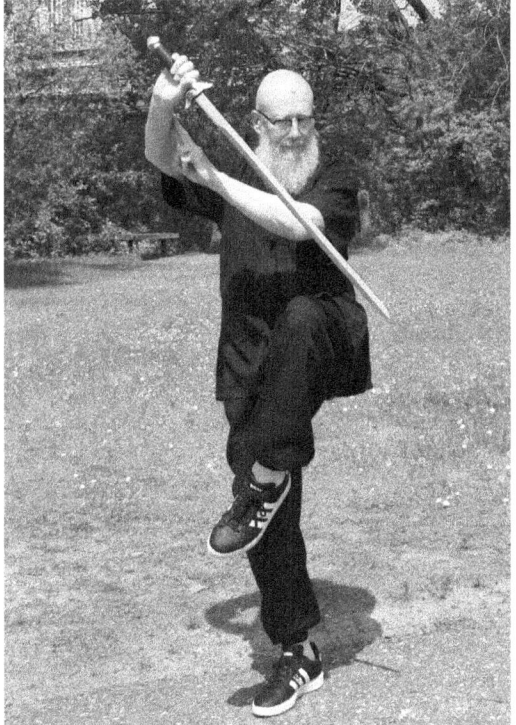

"Loyalty to a style or form keeps you from making changes for the better."

~ Grandmaster Wai-lun Choi

Appendix

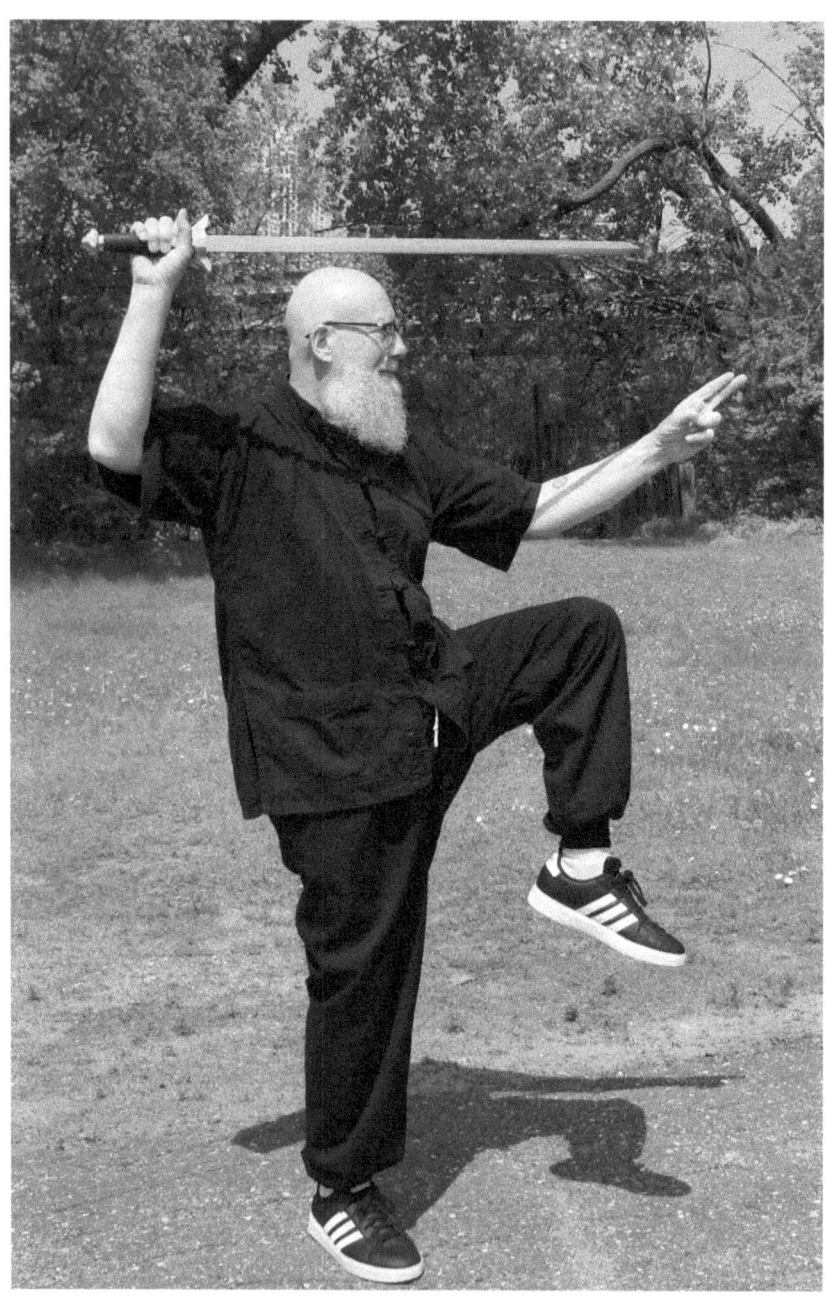

Why You Should Study T'ai-Chi

Joanne Von Blon; 7th Generation Lineage Holder and Founding Board of Directors Member of Twin Cities T'ai Chi Ch'uan, and Studio Patron, 2002

"Ray," I said, "what should I write for the anniversary?" He said, "Why don't you write what you would tell people who ask why they should take T'ai-Chi?" After 20 years of practice and at age 78, I can do that.

If they were young I would tell them that T'ai-Chi will improve their performance in any other sport they ever undertake. To be relaxed is to be fast and to be relaxed saves energy. I would tell them that T'ai-Chi is a magnificent fighting art and superb self-defense, but it takes a lot of training and they are lucky to start young.

I would add that the meditation practice would improve their concentration and lessen test anxieties. Finally, I would say that their friends would be curious and admire them for doing something a little different.

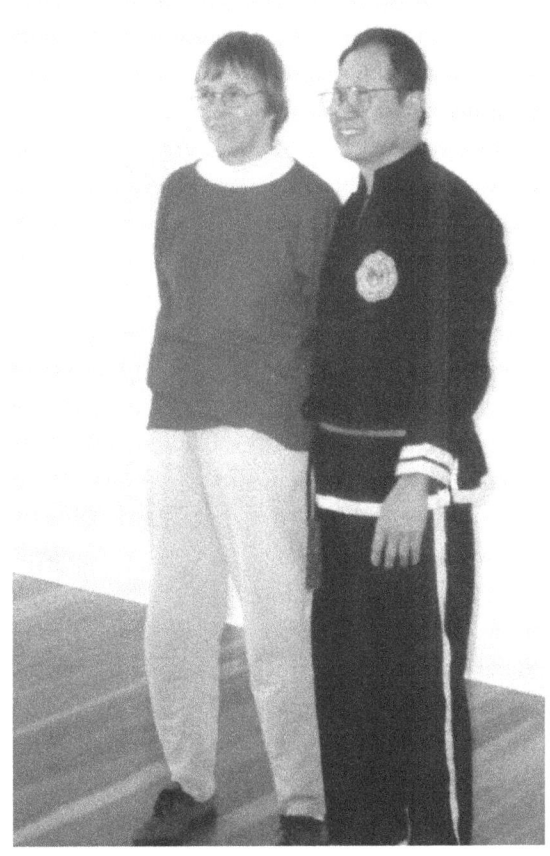

If they were closer to my age I would tell them that T'ai-Chi promises eternal Springtime, that we will carry good health into advanced old age. T'ai-Chi is moderate, safe exercise that engages every muscle group and works the mind and body as one entity. Because T'ai-Chi breathing trains the body to use oxygen more efficiently, the exercise is also aerobic. T'ai-Chi reduces stress, and stress is bad for our hearts.

Our balance will improve, lessening the likelihood of a fall. And if we should fall, our center of gravity has sunk and our relaxation response will make injury less likely. T'ai-Chi is a weight-bearing exercise that strengthens bones, lessening the danger of osteoporosis and a broken hip.

An added plus for Minnesota winters: the relaxation allows the blood to circulate through all the capillaries, keeping our hands and feet warmer. When we learn "reverse breathing" we warm up even faster.

For the majority of students in the middle age ranges, all of the above holds true and T'ai-Chi holds even more satisfactions. First, there is the discipline and fun of learning the Solo Form, something entirely new. This is followed, as we learn to relax, by the satisfaction of measurable progress. These epiphanies may be the best part of T'ai-Chi and they continue to happen from time to time for as long as we practice.

Those of us who go on to further study can learn sword, spear, cane and other weapons; we practice "pushing hands;" we learn the "two-person dance." Many of us begin to tutor other students, which adds to our own knowledge and pleasure. We meet the challenges of overcoming inevitable plateaus, and most importantly, the real joy and excitement of sudden insights, the knowledge that suddenly you did it right!

If any persons were still listening, I'd tell them two more things. One, that I treasure doing T'ai-Chi with and knowing an astounding diversity of men and women. And finally, I would say that in all their lives they will seldom meet a finer man, a better martial artist, or a funnier, more imaginative, or more creative teacher than mine.

~ Joanne

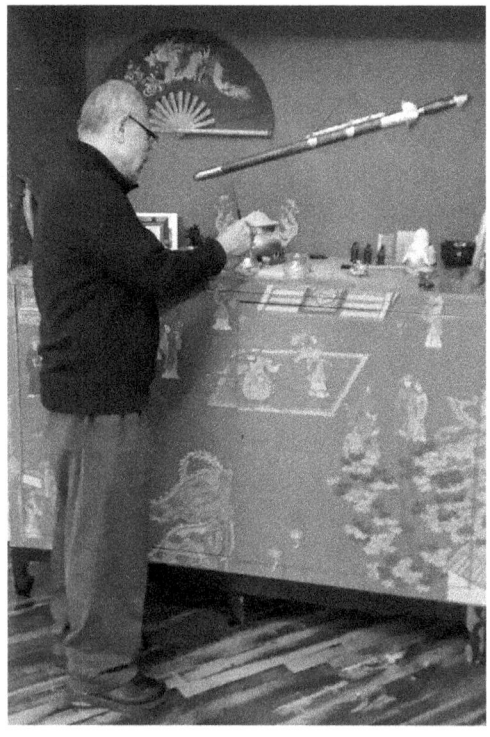

Push Hands: Just One Aspect of Self-Defense

By Ray Hayward
(first published in Tai-Chi Magazine, date??)

Is there too much emphasis on pushing hands? The answer to this question is yes. Pushing hands is only the second step of a four-step process we go through to acquire the art of T'ai Chi Ch'uan for self-defense. The first step is equilibrium. The second is pushing hands. The third is free-hand. The fourth is weapons training.

Now let me briefly explain each step so we can see what each has to contribute to our self-defense training.

The first step, equilibrium, is also called "getting a root." When we practice T'ai Chi Ch'uan, we must pay extra attention to our steps. When we step with our foot, it should be empty, then we should gradually shift our weight to that foot.

Achieving a Root Is Essential

In this way, we can fully exercise our legs and gain enough flexible strength to be able to "root." If you step with weight on both feet, you will be committing the mistake of "double-weighting" and will be taken far off the path to equilibrium.

When you have gained a root, no one can push you over, no matter what technique they use. You have the energy to resist, but won't, and can neutralize an opponent's energy because your waist can now obey your mind.

If you don't have a root, when you turn your waist to neutralize, you will fall over by your

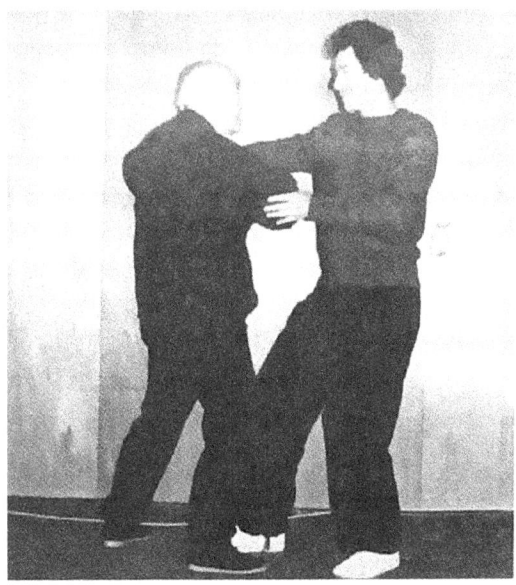

T.T. Liang, left, in elbow stroke with Ray Hayward.

action. Without a root, you won't be able to apply the subtle techniques of T'ai Chi Ch'uan. So, this can be considered the most important step.

The second step, pushing hands, can be divided into two parts. The first part is learning how to yield. This is for defense. We want to lose, not gain—small loss, small gain; big loss, big gain. When we are pushed, we don't resist.

Pushed 100 Times. Yield 100 Times

If we can't neutralize, we just fall over without a struggle. This is called "investing in loss," which rids us of our ego and fully exercises our legs to further develop our root.

Gradually, we will be able to neutralize and not let our opponent's energy come to our body. If we are pushed 100 times, we will yield 100 times, never losing balance. We are like a willow tree, bending 100 times in the wind. Our waist seems "boneless." Once you reach this stage, you can go on to learn the second part of pushing hands: counter-attack.

To counter-attack the opponent is not so easy. You must know the techniques of insubstantial and substantial, and the techniques of finding the center of gravity, and finding your opponent's defect position while maintaining your superior position.

You must also know the most effective line to push the opponent, and how to concentrate your energy in one direction while avoiding "double-weighting."

You must not collide with your opponent. You must know about all the kinds of energies, such as withdraw-attack energy, uprooting energy, "on the spot" energy, sudden energy, neutralizing energy, hearing energy, receiving energy, interpreting energy, and the sticking energy as used by the Yang family.

There are many more kinds of energy, but all of them come from using the whole body as one unit. If you don't have a 11 of these conditions before you counter-attack the opponent, you will fall into the error of "double-weighting" and only execute a "blind push." Only these techniques can be considered the true way of counter-attacking in T'ai Chi Ch'uan.

The Third Step

The third step, free-hand. can also be divided into two parts: da-lu and sparring sets. Da-lu is an advanced practice in which two people use the original 13 postures to attack and defend.

Da lu helps the practitioner to further understand the neutralizing, pushing, and striking techniques as well as how utilize the five steps and the eight directions. An example is the Yang family's da lu, which uses the techniques of roll back, push, shoulder, and slap, following the eight directions.

Wang Yen-nien's da lu uses ward-off, roll-back, push, and press against pull, split, elbow, and shoulder following an East-West direction.

The sparring sets, also called "miscellaneous combat," use the postures fran the solo form as well as auxiliary tech1iques to show how the principles of T'ai Chi Ch'uan are used to handle counter-punching and kicking attacks as well as pushing and grappling attacks.

Included in every posture are the three techniques of hua/neutralize, na/hold, and da/attack. The sets also teach how to "join" with an opponent, and how to "stick" with them so you can sense their intention You also review all the push hands techniques as well as learn how to "change steps" and "turn body." You learn various "folding" techniques as well as how to control your opponent.

Without learning the third step it will be difficult to engage in combat with opponents from other martial arts systems. It should be noted that my teacher, T. T. Liang, combined all the push hands, da lus and sparring sets into one form he calls the T'ai Chi two-person dance. By practicing one round of this form, which has 178 postures, students can cover all the aspects of the two-person training.

The fourth step, weapons training, is very important to the development of the intrinsic energy.

By practicing the empty hand forms, we are starting to develop the intrinsic ener-

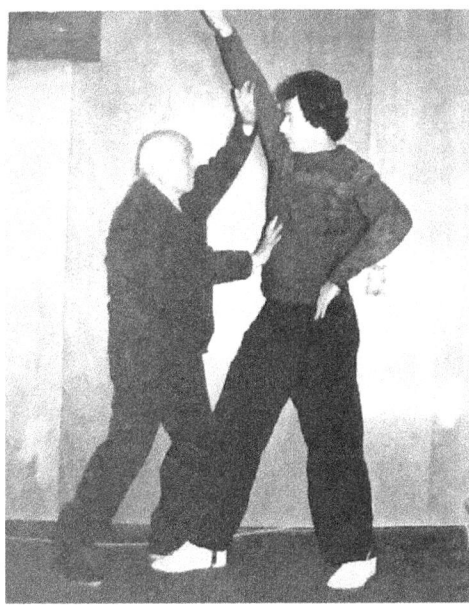

T. T. Liang uses Fair Lady at Shuttles on Ray Hayward.

119

gy, but by practicing with weapons we can fully develop our energy.

Most martial arts strike out with arm, which uses force from the bone. This force is exhaustible as well as detrimental to health. T'ai Chi Ch1uan uses the intrinsic energy which canes from the sinews and tendons of the whole body. The added weight of the weapons helps lo fully strengthen the sinews, which in turn strengthens the intrinsic energy.

When practicing empty-handed, we try to get our energy to our hands, but when using the weapons. We try to extend our energy to the very tip of the weapon. After practicing with weapons, we find it easier to get energy into our hands as well as an increased amount of energy at our command.

So, the purpose of weapon training is to fully develop and liberate our intrinsic energy. If you don't have this energy, you won't be able to apply the techniques of T'ai Chi Ch'uan and will never advance even to the lowest levels.

In conclusion, let me say that the reason some modern practitioners can't use their art for self-defense is because they haven't followed the correct procedure of learning and practicing.

Equal attention must be given to the four steps. Not one may be missing. Let us remember the Yang family and their disciples, who depended solely on T'ai Chi Ch'uan for their self-defense skills.

All the afore'llef1tioned information was told and taught to me by my master, Liang Tung-tsai. My deepest thanks go to him.

Ray Hayward teaches in Minneapolis, MN.

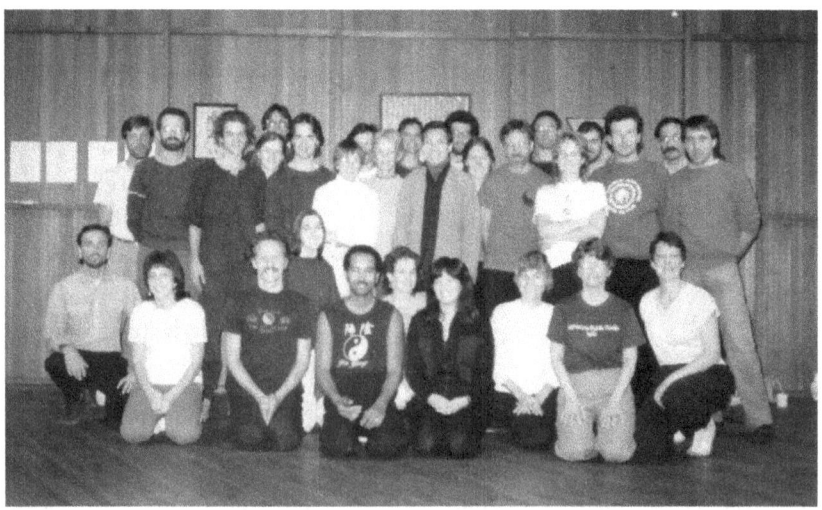

Grandmaster William C. C. Chen seminar, St Paul, 1985.

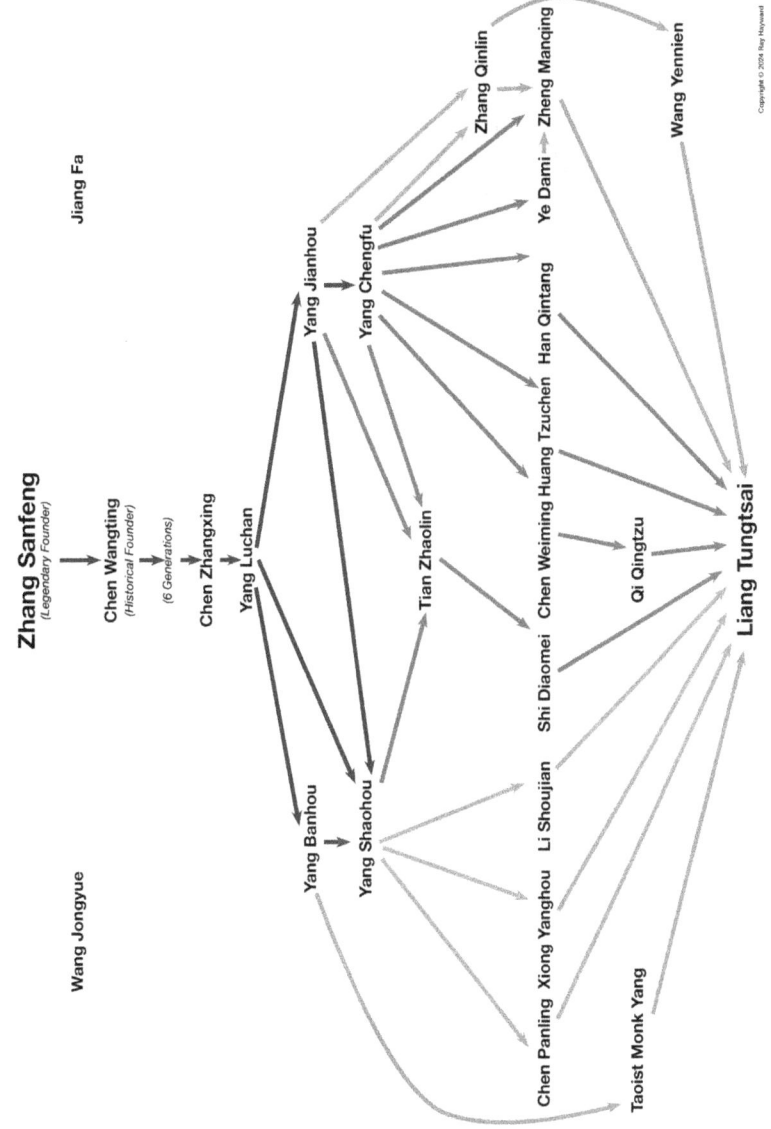

Joanne Von Blon 1924-2024

'(Joanne) Von Blon approached her own aging with a similar wit. "They used to say that if you did tai chi you'd live forever," she'd often say. "What was I thinking?" '

It is with profound gratitude and appreciation, the loss hasn't settled in yet, that I inform you of the passing of Joanne Von Blon. Joanne was one of my first students when I moved to Minnesota. She studied privately and in group classes and learned the complete Yang Style Taiji system. Joanne was my first disciple and a staunch supporter of me and my art. She and her husband Phil converted our school to a non-profit organization and her foundation supported us for many years. I talked to her on her 100th birthday this past March and congratulated her on reaching the highest level of immortality! Julie Cisler kept in close contact with Joanne all these years and was instrumental in scheduling visits and keeping her in the loop with all things Taiji.

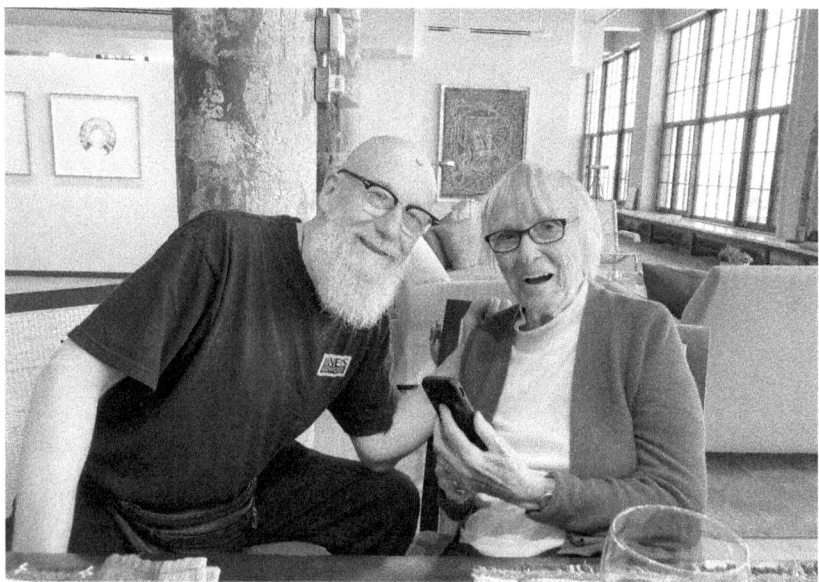

About the Authors

Margo Zi Yan began studying and practicing Taiji in the Minnesota spring of 2008. Since then, she has learned solo forms in Taiji, Sword, Sword with Tassel, Sabers, Staff, and Spear; along with studying other internal arts of Bagua, Xingyi, Luk Hop Bat Fa, meditation and Qigong. Additionally, areas of study are 2-person forms in San Shou, pushing hands, and Bagua. In 2018, she became an inner door student of Sifu Ray Hayward as a 7th-Generation lineage holder in Yang-Style T'ai Chi Ch'uan. Margo's lineage is Yang Lu-ch'an (Founder), Yang Chien-hou (2nd Generation), Yang Ch'eng-fu (3rd Generation), Zhang Man-ch'ing (4th Generation), Liang Tung-tsai (5th Generation), Sifu Ray Hayward (6th Generation). Her favorite Taiji movement is Parting Wild Horse's Mane and favorite Taiji place is in a park by the water.

Julie Cisler began her T'ai-Chi Ch'uan studies in 1986, while attending the University of South Dakota, learning the PRC Form under Sensei Richard Mesmer. In 1997, she met her current master, Sifu Ray Hayward (Shu-Kuang). She has continued her studies with Master Hayward to the present day. Julie received lineage from Sifu Hayward as a seventh-generation Yang-Style T'ai-Chi Ch'uan inner-door student in 2016, directly handed down from Master T. T. Liang and his teacher, professor Zheng Manqing. She has also had great privilege to study with Sifu Hayward's current teacher, Grandmaster Wai-lun Choi. Julie began teaching full-time in 2008, to pursue her passion for sharing T'ai-Chi, the 'Whole World's Exercise'. In addition to the T'ai-Chi solo form, she has also trained in T'ai-Chi weapons, Pushing-Hands, and Qigong. Julie has studied other martial arts including Baguazhang, Hsing-Yi Ch'uan, Liu Ho Ba Fa, Shaolin Kung-fu, Jook Lum Southern Praying Mantis, Tae Kwon Do, and Aikido.

Teacher, writer, content creator, martial artist, and spiritual seeker, **Ray Hayward (Shu-Kuang)** has studied with some of the highest-level martial art masters and spiritual teachers in the world including Master T.T. Liang, Grandmaster Wai-lun Choi, Judge

David Sinclair Bouschor, and Chosen Chief Philip Carr-Gomm.

Ray began his health maintenance and martial arts training in 1973, eventually studying Kenpo Karate, Ng Cho Kuen, and Jiu-Jitsu with Sensei John Duncan. In 1977, Ray met and began study with Master T.T. Liang in Boston. Ray learned the complete Yang Style Taiji Quan system from Master Liang, as well as Praying Mantis, Qigong, Taoist Meditation, Qinna, Wudang Sword and various weapons. In 1984, Ray moved to Minnesota to continue studying with Master Liang. In 1988, Ray Hayward passed through a formal ceremony to become an inner-door disciple of Master T.T. Liang.

He studied Northern 7-Star Praying Mantis and Eagle Claw with Sifu Lo Man-biu, and Bagua Zhang, Xingyi Quan, Chen Style Taiji, Qinna, and weapons from Dr. Leung Kay-chi. Ray learned Taoist Meditation, Qigong, 5 Animal Frolics, and Taiji Ruler from Masters Paul B. Gallagher and Kenneth Cohen.

Other teachers include Master William C.C. Chen, Master B.P. Chan, Mr. Heintz Rottmann, and Shifu Li Wang. Ray currently studies Modern Tactical Martial Arts with Master Rob Jones, and the breathwork of Wim Hof, Patrick McGowen, and Stig Severinsen.

To round out and finish his martial arts studies, Ray learned the complete systems of Xingyi Quan, Bagua Zhang, Yiquan, and Wudang Sword from Grandmaster Wai-lun Choi. Ray also studied Luk Hop Bat Fat, Taiji, Lama, Qinna, Qigong, Taoist Meditation, and basic TCM traumatology with Master Choi.

With a deep interest in spirituality and meditation, Ray has explored many Eastern religions, focusing on Taoism and Sufism. He has also studied Hypnotherapy, Psychology, and is certified in the Healing Tao System. For the past twenty-five years, Ray has made extensive research and study concerning the Western Mysteries, including Alchemy, Freemasonry, the Knights Templar, the Rosicrucians, Druidry, Celtic history, and Rosslyn Chapel, studying with such masters as PGM David Sinclair Bouschor, WB Joseph Lang, REPGC Charles W. Nelson, and PCC Philip Carr-Gomm. In 2010, Ray became a Druid Graduate in the Order of Bards, Ovates, and Druids.

Ray Hayward approaches teaching through many modalities: in person classes, zoom classes, books, instructional videos, blogs, vlogs, seminars, workshops, podcasts, retreats, YouTube, Patreon, and in private consultation. Ray has taught martial arts and meditation to hundreds of people, particularly Taiji Quan, as a way to gain health, peace of mind, physical confidence, and a state of well-being. He teaches martial arts to empower, not overpower, others.

"Forty-seven years is a short time when exploring the mysteries and experiencing the benefits of the art of Taiij Quan."
~ Ray Hayward

Contact Information

Margo Zi Yan
YouTube: www.youtube.com/@purpleswallowartsbyziyan6991
Website: https://purpleswallowarts.com/
Email: ziyan.purpleswallow8@gmail.com

Julie Cisler
Mindful Motion Tai-Chi Academy email: mindfulmotiontaichi@gmail.com
Other email: juliecisler13@hotmail.com

Ray Hayward
Blog: rayhayward.com
Patreon: patreon.com/rayhayward
YouTube: Ray Hayward, the Inspired Teacher
Facebook: Mindful Motion Tai-Chi Academy
Lulu Books: lulu.com/spotlight/Ray_Hayward